Advance Praise for
Cancer Just Is: Convictions of a
20-Something Exploring His Illness,
Faith & Culture

In this gripping narrative, Morgan Bolt speaks with such an honest, eloquent, and compelling voice that it must join the chorus of America's most memorable literary narrators. But instead of rafting the Mississippi River, exploring the West, or wandering New York, Bolt's journey takes him into the harrowing clinical corridors of a young cancer patient prematurely confronting death. His powerful account of that pilgrimage, however, is a bittersweet celebration of a life, told with disarming humor, unflinching candor, and a remarkable wisdom and faith that will be a gift to all who listen.

—Kerry Temple
Editor of *Notre Dame Magazine*
Author of *Back to Earth: A Backpacker's Journey into Self and Soul*

Smyth & Helwys Publishing, Inc.
6316 Peake Road
Macon, Georgia 31210-3960
1-800-747-3016

Library of Congress Cataloging-in-Publication Data

CIP Information on file

CANCER JUST IS

CONVICTIONS OF A

20-SOMETHING EXPLORING

HIS ILLNESS, FAITH & CULTURE

Morgan J. Bolt

Also by Morgan J. Bolt

The Tamyth Trilogy:
The Rise of Gnurlbane
Westerly
Return to Rythka

The Favored

To all who face pediatric cancer

Acknowledgments

The outpouring of love and support, from people I have known my whole life and some whom I have never once met in person, has been encouraging beyond description, and I cannot thank everyone enough for the dozens of ways they have shown exceptional generosity to us throughout the last few years. There are far too many people on similar journeys without the incredible support network my wife and I enjoy. I am deeply thankful for the countless blessings that enrich my life. The care package financial gifts, sharing of a beautiful home on the Finger Lakes, visits, thoughtful emails, and so much more have made all the difference the last four years. So to those who gave generously of your time, letters, money, gifts, cards, and more, thank you.

I want to thank those who support the Ronald McDonald House, whether in New York, in your own hometowns, or as an organization as a whole. Because of your generosity, my wife and I had a true home away from home, and experienced a range of activities otherwise quite beyond our reach. I cannot say enough good things about the Ronald, the people who work there, and the many volunteers who make it feel like home.

If you donate blood regularly or even occasionally, thank you.

I also can't thank the role models I've had in New York City enough, be they two years old or twenty, for showing me what a cancer patient is, is not, and can be. I've not been one to reach out on message boards or support groups, but I have nonetheless received strength and encouragement from others going through treatment as well, and for that I will always be grateful.

To all the medical workers who have worked with me over the years, thank you. Starting on day one with the doctor at the urgent care center who recommended a PET scan, to the nurses we've gotten to know at Sloan

Kettering that Christina and I can honestly count as friends, to my radiologist, surgeon, and oncologists, your knowledge, compassion, and skill has made all the difference. From researching other treatment options, helping me make the best decisions with limited options, to facilitating my travels even when my health made traveling extremely difficult, my oncologist and several great RNs have been invaluable and wonderful beyond what I could ever reasonably expect. Extra thanks are due to my surgeon, for all your careful work, your kindness, and your willingness to come in at 6 a.m. to drain fluid from my abdomen on a Sunday morning when you should have been sleeping in.

I am immensely grateful for today's level of knowledge about cancer, for the ever-improving treatment regimens available, and for the affordable access to this care that I've enjoyed. That my wife and I could quit our jobs and devote ourselves to getting me the best care possible while I remained under my parents' health insurance was an enormous blessing. Many people don't have that kind of option, and many families are split by work back home and hospital stays elsewhere and face even more uncertainty than I ever did about the future of their healthcare.

I remain forever grateful to those who have helped with my writing endeavors, starting with my oldest sister, Elyssa, who has been onboard reviewing my first drafts for as long as I have been writing. I want to extend a huge thank you to my writing mentor, Bill Russell, who I was matched with through Sloan Kettering's Visible Ink writing mentorship program, as well as everyone in the Corning Area Writer's Group. Beyond your critiques, having a couple hours a week to escape my cancer and immerse myself in a range of wonderful writing has been a real highlight of the past year for me. Thank you also to Kerry Temple at *Notre Dame Magazine* for believing in my writing when I was starting not to, and thank you as well to Rob Lee, who wrote the foreword for this book. You got me in touch with a publisher right after I got the worst PET scan of my life and I had just about given up on ever publishing this book. Writing, editing, and publishing are a path that cannot be traveled alone, so once again, thank you to everyone who has supported and enabled my writing the last four years.

To my extended family, thank you for everything. The care packages, the stroopwafels, the visits, emails, cards, phone calls, Facebook messages, and more have been such a blessing, and I will always be grateful for your love.

To my in-laws: you have truly outdone yourselves with your generous support and encouragement. You have opened your home and your hearts and made me feel like a welcome addition to your family. It has been such a blessing to get to experience new sides of you and to see that many of the qualities I love about Christina are shared by all of you. And Rachel, you're a pretty great third wheel to have tag along on our travels (cheeky smile emoji).

I really cannot say enough good things about my parents, who have gone above and beyond, initially researching which hospital I should go to for treatment and remaining supportive and involved ever since. You've helped make sure I have health insurance, given Christina and me a third of your house to live in, and, most impressively, found that tricky balance between caring for your child and letting me be an adult and live as normal a life as possible. Your support has been such a blessing to me, and I'm thankful for the ways cancer has drawn us closer.

I have been fortunate to grow closer to my three wonderful siblings as well during the last few years. You have all made impressive efforts to spend as much time with me as possible, visiting from afar more frequently than I'd have thought possible and helping in so many different ways. Through the hours spent playing and fighting over board games like Settlers of Catan and Power Grid, visiting theme parks, and just hanging out together, we've become better friends now than ever before, and I will treasure all three of you forever.

Christina, you don't get enough appreciation and I know saying "thank you" here doesn't make up for that, but thank you. You have modeled strength, perseverance, and fierce love unmatched by anyone else on this journey. I don't know how you've managed to be both a caretaker and a wife, to balance the realities of our situation with life as we want it to be, but you have as well as humanly possible, certainly better than I ever could have in your place. For everything you do and everything you are, thank you.

Contents

Foreword
by Rob Lee

I wonder if you're like me, if you've been asking lately where God is amidst the fray of life. I first encountered Morgan on Twitter; amidst the fray of my Twitter followers, he stuck out as a deep thinker and an even better theologian. We exchanged some messages, and he communicated his dream: he wanted to be a published author. I did what I could to get him connected to the right people, and we were able to make that happen. Then I received a copy of the book, and I found the answer to my question: God is right here. God is right now. Most importantly, God is love.

This book is not an easy read. If you're looking for theological platitudes and superficial half-truths, look elsewhere. But if you're looking for deep answers to life's questions, to the intricacies of God and God's presence in sickness and health, then this book is for you. Morgan has poured his whole heart and soul into this work, and it will be part of his legacy even after he has left this life for the next.

So if the news of the day is too grim, if life is weighing you down, be strong like Morgan has been and reflect on the love and grace of God. Sam Wells, my favorite theologian, says, "If it can't be happy, make it beautiful." Nothing about Morgan's prognosis is happy—but his response to it has been remarkably beautiful, full of the hope extended to him by his Creator. It reminds me of the Statement of Faith from the United Church of Canada: "In life, in death, in life beyond death, we are not alone, God is with us."

Friends, this book is a testament to the love and grace of God. I hope you will read it and find there is more to life than meets the eye. And when Morgan is commended to God, this will be the hope we hold onto.

I'm better off because I encountered this book, and you will be too. Read it, consume it, and hold on to that love. For the love that made you will indeed be the love that brings you, and all of us, home.

—Rob
The Reverend Robert W. Lee, IV

Prologue

On September 19, 2018, two days after turning twenty-seven, I got the worst scan results of my life. The clinical trial I had been on the last nine weeks wasn't doing anything, and instead my cancer had suddenly started to spread exponentially. I had lesions lighting up in my liver, which had always been clear of disease previously, and dozens of other nodes lay scattered from my pelvis into my neck. My cancer has always been incurable, but for nearly four years it had been a managed, chronic condition. Not anymore. Today I'm on a low-dose chemotherapy that consists of a couple pills each evening, hoping it buys me a little more time than I'd otherwise get, but realistically I'm looking at weeks to months until my cancer kills me. For now I feel mostly all right, just tired and worn down. I use a walker now, cannot stand for more than a brief moment, and require a handful of enzyme supplements to digest food. The only real question I have now is how my cancer will kill me, whether through respiratory, cardiac, digestive, or some less foreseeable trouble. It's likely that by the time you're reading this, we'll know the answer to that question.

Such is life.

Because such is life, because this sort of thing happens, because so many people have given me their own theories about why this sort of thing happens, and because I tend to disagree with just about everyone on that subject, I decided to write this book.

Before we dive in, I think it would be helpful for me to take a step back and explain what this book is and is not. It's a reflection on my own experiences with cancer, sure, but I hope it is much more than that. My interest in cancer before I was diagnosed with the disease was pretty close to zero, and if anything that interest has decreased in the years since then. I don't enjoy cancer memoir as a genre, and this book isn't designed to be one. Instead, it's a theological exploration of suffering through the lens of my own experiences with cancer—which has been in many ways an incredibly privileged experience, despite the terribleness of my disease. This book is ultimately about faith and what it means to have hope, even if that hope may not be for anything in this world. It's about God as I know God, as I've experienced God, as I love God, and as I understand God in light of my cancer.

If that sounds like highly contextual theology, well, it is. All theology is contextual, after all, and mine is no different. I don't have any formal theological or philosophical training. I don't have all the right answers. I may not even be asking the right questions. I merely seek to present how my experiences with cancer have—and have not—shaped my experience of God.

—Morgan J. Bolt
October 10, 2018

Chapter 1

Cancer Is Not Evil

When I vomited two mornings straight, I knew something was amiss. Christina, my wife, said I needed to call off work and have a doctor look at me. So I went to an urgent care center where a wonderful, life-saving doctor whose name I do not recall spent about three seconds looking me over before telling me I had some "large, very concerning masses" in my abdomen and needed a PET scan as soon as possible. Like, in an hour or two. He wrote it all down on a sticky note for me and printed off directions to the nearest hospital, which was great because I had no idea where any hospitals were in the Harrisburg, Pennsylvania, area; I had only lived there while going to college and had graduated just a few months before. That doctor was the first in a long procession of people who saved my life over the next few years. I owe my life to his promptness and willingness to convey the severity of my condition. I wish I knew his name.

I drove to the closest hospital, went in the wrong entrance, and was told by a pair of friendly custodians how to get to the emergency room. There I gave the receptionist the sticky note that the doctor at urgent care had signed to expedite the process, and they took me to a back room right away. I turned on a football game and drank my first liter of contrast, which, as I understand it, is radioactive sugar water that tastes worse the more you drink. I would drink many more liters of the stuff in the coming years, but of course at the time I did not know that. All I recall thinking then was that if I had cancer, I'd simply have to beat it. And also, the Indianapolis Colts defense needed some work, giving up fifty-one points to the Pittsburgh Steelers.

After my first set of PET/CT scans, which involved taking a nap on a surprisingly comfortable plank while slowly being fed through the middle of a giant, donut-shaped machine, my wife Christina joined me, having gotten off work early once it became clear that something was seriously amiss. As one doctor put it, "If you were old . . . *eh*. But you're young, so we'll fight this thing with everything we can." I personally appreciated that. Better to have too morbid a picture painted early on than to be told everything will be fine and get blindsided with bad news after the test results are finalized.

The PET/CT scans showed multiple large masses from my pelvis to my diaphragm. I threw up in the mornings because, not unlike what happens during pregnancy, my organs were being pushed around and displaced by the thing growing inside my belly—a belly that now seemed obviously larger than normal. Before, I had simply attributed the size to marrying a fantastic cook the previous year. The rapidly assembling team of doctors assigned to me, some from specialties I had never heard of, scheduled a biopsy for the following morning. That team constitutes the next group of life-savers I am forever indebted to; it is in part thanks to the cooperation of that group of doctors—residents, fellows, an oncologist, a radiologist, and a bariatric weight-loss surgeon—that I am here today writing this book. They pooled their collective knowledge, decided what needed to be figured out next, and told us what major hospitals to research in the meantime.

It took more than a week for the biopsy results to come back, as they had to send my tissue sample to the Mayo Clinic to figure out what was growing inside me. My parents arrived from Corning, New York, and we set to work researching kinds of cancer, types of treatments, and hospitals that deal with rare cancers. Well, my parents and wife did. I only recall watching the BBC's *Sherlock* and eating a ton of candy, since Halloween was just a few days back and everything was on clearance.

First we thought I might have to drive the forty-five minutes or so to the hospital in Hershey. Then it seemed that the hour-and-a-half drive to Johns Hopkins might be my new commute. We started to wonder about the implications for our jobs and whether we might be home only on weekends—or even have to move. We had no idea what level of impact this cancer—if it was indeed cancer—might have on our lives.

Then we met with the bariatric surgeon, who said an official diagnosis would take a couple more days, but it looked like something called desmoplastic small round cell tumors (DSRCT), a soft-tissue sarcoma that's classified as a pediatric cancer. There is little information available on DSRCT, and much of it may not be entirely accurate. But according to Wikipedia—which the surgeon we met with had to turn to since he, like most doctors, had never heard of DSRCT—a mere 15 percent of people with this type of cancer are still alive five years after diagnosis. Only two hospitals in the country and in fact the world really deal with it, at least with any efficacy. We (my parents and wife) did more research on treatments, hospitals, and just how serious and life-altering this diagnosis would be. For my part, I made a lot of progress in "Real Racing 3," a car racing game on my phone.

Then the major, ineluctable changes to our lives began. It became clear that my treatment would last at least a year, involving too many procedures to make it feasible to work. So Christina quit both of her jobs even as she was in the middle of getting a promotion at one of them. She had found her niche working as an activities associate at a continuing care center, helping plan and run programs for residents with early-stage dementia. I quit both of my part-time jobs as well. I had greatly enjoyed working at a ski resort just fifteen minutes from our townhouse, and Christina and I had made good use of the free skiing and snowboarding perks it provided. More seriously, just one month earlier I had begun work as a teaching assistant, helping students who needed extra attention to excel in school. It was an incredibly rewarding job, which made for a heart-wrenching round of goodbyes to the kids I had worked with for far too short a time. Christina and I also went through our stuff and got everything ready to move into my parents' basement in New York. Fortunately, they have an in-law suite with a bathroom, kitchen, living room, and bedroom, so it's much better than it sounds.

The next week or so passed in a blur that I scarcely remember and don't care to try to recall in detail. I didn't keep a journal and I hadn't started blogging yet, but I can piece together some snapshots of that time with a little help. It's enough to convey the main idea of what went on.

We decided I should go to Memorial Sloan Kettering Cancer Center in New York City, since they had oncologists familiar with DSRCT, two surgeons willing to operate on people with DSRCT, and a doctor working on an experimental radio-immunotherapy trial. I remember my dad using choice words on the phone to get my biopsy sent to Sloan Kettering in time for my first appointment. For some reason, the sample went from Mayo Clinic to Johns Hopkins instead of Sloan Kettering, but with some persuasion from my dad it got to Sloan Kettering in time for the doctors there to review my results before they met me.

Our landlord let us out of our lease early without a fuss, and a kind bunch of other people moved us out of our townhouse and into my parents' house. I remember eating Domino's pizza in a Super 8 motel in

New Jersey the night before my first meet-and-greet with the doctors at Sloan Kettering, silently wondering if that would be the last time I'd eat a proper meal.

The first day at Sloan Kettering stands out in my mind more clearly than any other day around this time. We met with enough different doctors that I quickly lost track of who specialized in what. My new main oncologist asked if I wanted a rundown of all the types of chemotherapy they had planned and their side effects, so of course I said yes. After about twenty minutes, the differences started to blur together, but I wanted to know what I was facing. Next, I had a slew of scans: PET, CT, MRI. They also did another scan, the name of which I've long forgotten, that mapped how well my kidneys were draining. My first scan had showed that one of my kidneys was a little inflamed and the associated ureter—the tube that drains your kidneys into your bladder—might be pinched by tumors, and this follow-up test seemed to confirm that. I had other tests too, but they weren't as lengthy and I don't remember them anymore.

My wife and I drove back home, a little shell-shocked, and found ourselves stuck at a tollbooth that charged one dollar. Neither of us had any cash. In some ways, that was the lowest point of my life, though really it shouldn't even crack the top-ten list with everything I've been through. Yet somehow, the fact that there had been no toll heading eastbound but there was one returning westward, coupled with the ridiculousness of not having even one dollar on us, along with the booth's inability to accept debit or credit cards, made it seem like the end of the world. Coming from our first glimpse at what would soon be our new life in the pediatric cancer ward didn't help either. After trying to explain our situation to a toll road employee who, I thought, said to just drive through and not worry about paying, we went home only to receive a bill for one dollar in the mail a week later. We have an EZ pass transponder now.

A couple days later, I had my first surgery, a planned forty-five minutes that ended up running into the four-hour neighborhood. They placed my double-lumen mediport, a device in my chest just under my skin that allows for easier IV access and infusions of chemotherapy without damaging my skin and veins. They also put stents in both ureters, which was an unexpectedly difficult process, thanks to the tumors pinching them, but my superbly talented surgeon got them installed. He's another person I owe my life to, and I'm sure I'll mention him many, many more times in this book. I don't know why it took four hours to install these stents, and I don't really need to. I know they ran into complications and had to try a couple different sizes to get them in place, but eventually the surgery team prevailed. I didn't have to have a nephrostomy tube—basically a reroute of my urinary tract from my kidney out through my back into a plastic bag like they said was a possibility—so that was a win. I peed fire for a few days, but it was worth saving my kidneys and maintaining the ability to urinate conventionally.

I woke up from that surgery vomiting as I was wheeled out of the operating room, which my anesthesia-addled mind knew was bad but couldn't figure out why. I woke up again a little later in the recovery room, feeling a trifle less terrible, though I still threw up a couple more times before the anti-nausea meds kicked in. I remember thinking that this wasn't worth it if it only bought me a few extra weeks, so I needed to keep going a while longer.

A week or so later I started chemo, a reportedly "easy," relatively low-dose regimen that was part of an experimental protocol to see if the combination of drugs was, as my oncologist put it, "tolerable" for people with DSRCT to start on before going to the more standard-protocol chemo regimens. If I'm reading between the lines correctly, that means people don't go downhill any quicker on this experimental regimen than they would otherwise. Comforting.

On this supposedly easy and tolerable chemo, I was violently ill, got a bacterial infection called C. diff (short for clostridium difficile infection), barely ate, and went down to my lowest weight ever, some sixty pounds less than what I was before I started treatment, none of which I needed to lose. Other than the several pounds of tumor, of course. And maybe about ten pounds or so that I'd gained in college. By any reckoning, though, there's no way someone with my six-foot-two frame should weigh in the low 150s. It was perhaps the roughest month or two of my life. I was glad to leave it behind me.

Clearly, my cancer has necessitated a lot of treatment and medical attention, none of it particularly pleasant. But I have almost never felt uneasy about it, and never for more than a fleeting moment. I know I can't speak for anyone else on this journey with me, but I have only rarely felt truly unsettled about it. Have I looked forward to the various toxins of chemotherapy? Hardly. Have I been excited when surgeons describe an upcoming procedure and its recovery process? Not exactly. I've been nervous about radiation, my next surgery, impending scans, and new regimens of chemotherapy. But am I unsettled? Am I shaken and rattled to my core? Have I fallen apart and questioned the fairness of life? No.

That's a large part of why I'm writing this book. Not to give all the answers to life's tough questions—I certainly don't have them—but simply to share how my perspectives and beliefs helped me through a truly difficult, trying phase of life. Most of how I've remained largely upbeat and unfazed through my grueling treatments has been because of my faith and how it compels me to regard the world. If my beliefs have helped me through an immensely difficult time, then perhaps others might find some value in them as they face difficulties and struggles.

I'd like to insert a disclaimer about myself: I'm a bit weird. They say don't sweat the small things in life, but I disagree. That might be sage advice for many, and I understand the theory; don't stress over the little things that really don't mean much, and your life will likely contain far less angst. Keeping minor inconveniences in perspective is certainly healthy, and building a lifestyle where molehills are left as molehills is easier on you and the people around you. I'm sure it works for lots of people, but it doesn't really work for me.

I *like* to sweat the small things in life. I like to overreact to little annoyances, like a wrinkle in my shirt that lies uncomfortably against my back, or when I feel too hot, or when someone doesn't drive the way I think they should, or any number of equally trivial, mildly bothersome conditions. Most of the things I like to get worked up over have to do with being physically uncomfortable. They're silly things, and I know it's silly to get upset over them. That's part of the fun, though. If my shirt is wrinkled, I freak out, and then I make fun of myself for freaking out. Freaking out about little things gives me a necessary outlet for expressing stress and frustration, and laughing at myself for getting worked up about minor inconveniences helps me keep them in perspective and remember that they are indeed meaningless. Regardless of how meaningless they are, this is a helpful, useful practice for me.

By stressing out and sweating the small stuff, I feel much freer to remain calm when it comes to serious matters. Everyone has stress, and everyone needs to express frustrations and let off steam. Either we vent our frustrations in healthy ways or we eventually erupt. I typically choose to vent several times a day, never for very long and never over anything important. It works for me at least most of the time, when it doesn't annoy everyone around me. But I find it helpful to vent about little issues and to stay at ease and focus on what needs to be done when it comes to serious problems. I'd rather have the presence of mind and the clarity to react in the best possible way if I found myself in an impending car crash or with, say, a morbid cancer diagnosis. I wouldn't want to freak out and panic if my ability to stay calm and drive well in an emergency situation could help minimize damage and injury. I wouldn't want to worry myself to death over my low chances of surviving cancer. So I don't. Maintaining a steady supply of minor annoyances to stress about whenever I need to vent is helpful and mostly frees me of stress when it comes to the real problems in life.

I certainly cannot—or at least should not—give myself too much credit for this. By nature I am laid back, and, by whatever combination of nature and nurture, I tend not to worry about much at all. I'm not anxious or stressed by default, and I often live in a world where I happily ignore problems as much as I can and enjoy life despite what might be going wrong around me. This can be problematic when weightier issues require my attention, like getting a job or keeping track of literally anything my wife asks me to do for us or making important decisions. But it has also saved me and the people around me a world of stress throughout the past four years. I took my diagnosis better than anyone else involved in my life. Nobody had to worry about keeping me cheerful or relatively happy. Actually, I've had to comfort people far more than they've had to comfort me.

I cannot say for certain that my habit of worrying over minor annoyances, giving me a healthy outlet to vent my frustrations, is how I've managed to stay calm and mostly happy since my diagnosis. Nor do I suggest that everyone try worrying about every little thing in an attempt to live a more stress-free life. I do think that it is worth reconsidering the adage, though. Sometimes sweating the small stuff is freeing, constructive, and healthy. It helps me stay calm and focused when the big stuff comes my way.

The most significant source of strength I draw from as I deal with cancer, however, is not some coping mechanism that comes naturally to me. I don't have three keys for stress-free living to offer my readers. Instead, the most important, most helpful sources of inspiration and strength for me have been my beliefs about God and the way God's world works. I'll explore those here and in the coming chapters.

My first observation is that *cancer is not evil.*

This statement may seem shocking, especially coming from someone who has been profoundly affected by the disease, but I find it to be true. I want to begin by discussing evil—what it is and what it isn't. To do that, I need to address one of the most widely asked and poorly answered questions in human history: "Why does evil exist?"

This question can be framed in a myriad of ways. "Why do bad things happen to good people?" and "How could an all-knowing, all-loving, and all-powerful God allow evil?" are two of the most common ways to phrase this query. The book of Job, probably my favorite book in the Bible, says much about this subject, and I'll get into that in chapter 2. Right now, I want to dissect this common question because it actually contains two questions in one.

When people ask why evil exists, they typically wonder why human beings are allowed to commit evil acts. Why do murder and warfare happen? Why is there so much hatred in the world? As I see it, a world in which people have the ability to choose to love or hate is better than one in which people are not free to choose anything and are bound by the only possible course of action available to them. God could have made a world where people are programmed never to do evil, but in such a world we would not be free to choose love over hate. In such a world there would be no point to any of our actions, no reason to think or try to do what is right. We would be like marionettes. God would pull all the strings, and there would be no reason or even possibility for us to share God's love. That, in my opinion, is why people are allowed to do bad things.

That doesn't particularly pertain to cancer, though. Cancer brings up the second part of the question: Why do bad things just happen? For example, why do children get cancer for no real reason? Why do hurricanes, avalanches, and falling tree branches kill people? Why are these kinds of "evil" allowed? Well, because they aren't actually evil. We simply don't like them.

I don't think cancer is any more evil than weather, or mountains, or trees, or any other part of this world that can and does kill people. Cancer is simply part of life on this good earth. Sure, it causes suffering and death. So do storms, avalanches, and falling tree limbs. As far as I am aware, nobody claims that clouds, snowy peaks, or aged trees are inherently evil, no matter the fury of the hurricane, the power of the snow that roars down a slope, or the heft of the trunk that crashes down on a home. It would be bizarre to say that a natural process or event has moral value of any kind. Calling cancer evil, then, seems strange. Cancer does not have a conscience. It cannot decide to be good or evil. It merely is.

Some people may say that there's a difference. Weather, mountains, trees—these can all be beautiful or useful, or even both. These can be good! Well, no. Not in a moral sense of the word "good." They may be to our liking at times, but that does not make them good. Rather, they simply are. On the other side of that coin, people may hate cancer, but that alone does not make it evil. Cancer may bring only suffering and death, yes. But cell division keeps us all alive. It allows us to grow and heal. And what is cancer if not a hurricane of cell division? Cancer, then, is no more evil—or good—than any other part of this incredible and dynamic world in which we live. When natural events like the weather or cell division suit us, we like them. When they cause strife, we hate them. But they are not good when they make us comfortable or evil when they kill us. They just are.

Jesus expressed much the same idea. Tucked away in the Sermon on the Mount is a clear, concise explanation of how the world works, an explanation that too often remains overlooked. Jesus, when imploring his followers to love even their own enemies, says that God "makes the sun rise on the evil and on the good, and sends rain on the righteous and on the unrighteous" (Matt 5:45). In context, Jesus is talking about the need to love everyone, just as God blesses everyone with sunrises and nurturing rains. But there's more here for us to unpack. This isn't merely an imperative that we love even those who do not love us so that we can be more like God. It also reveals an important truth about God and the way God made the world. This world, Jesus says, rains and shines on the righteous and the unrighteous—on the people who love God and on those who despise God.

Interestingly, righteous and unrighteous as well as sunshine and rain are pairs of opposites that, as I recall from my "Encountering the Old Testament" Bible 203 class in college, imply the existence of "everything in between." To paraphrase, people ranging from good to bad all get weather ranging from good to bad more or less equally. It's important to remember that rain and shine aren't inherently good or bad. Too much or too little of either causes flooding or droughts.

The lesson here is profound. Jesus essentially states that God does not discriminate regarding who receives what from the natural systems of this world. Righteous or not, you will experience both rain and shine and every-thing in between. Events that seem good or bad happen to people who appear good or bad almost randomly, and making sense of what or who is good or bad and why such occurrences happen is a guessing game not worth playing (see more in chapter 2). The natural processes of this world simply function as God created them to function, and whether or not we always like them is irrelevant. Sometimes their effects will be unpleasant. While we might even call them evil, attaching such a moral attribute to them is useless. They just are. They simply occur.

The next logical question is why God would make a world like that. Why would God make a world with systems that can kill us? Why is weather allowed to become so extreme that it threatens human lives? Why does snow layer so unstably that it rages down mountainsides? Why are trees allowed to break and crash to earth?

This goes back to an idea I remember first pondering when I was five or six. As a child, I wondered if, in the Garden of Eden, the first humans were allowed to swat mosquitoes that bit them. One answer I heard then was that mosquitoes didn't evolve the ability or the need to drink blood until after the Fall. Which solved that problem, I guess, but it led to another question. What if I accidentally killed a bug in Eden? What if I breathed on one or stepped on it without meaning to? Then I started to expand on that idea. Could I run with scissors in the Garden of Eden? Like so many other children, I was told more than once not to do this very thing, since it is obviously dangerous, and it got me wondering. Could I climb trees in the Garden of Eden? No one can climb a tree without some risk of falling and becoming injured or even killed.

The more I've thought about it over the years, the more I've realized something fundamental about this material world: death is a risk inherent in any action we take. We can't walk—or bike, wheelchair, drive, take a train, or fly—anywhere without risking killing insects that we may not even be able to see, not to mention risking that we ourselves may die in some kind of accident. We can't wash our hands without killing germs. Even if we eat only the parts of plants that they can live without and regrow, we cannot do so without risking the deaths of microorganisms and even larger insects that might live on those plants. In fact, we cannot do anything at all without our actions potentially harming something, be it another living thing or ourselves. We could sit completely still forever, interacting with as little as possible, but we would die of dehydration in a few short days— and we'd still risk killing airborne bugs and microbes simply by breathing. Death, then, is a condition necessary to our ability to exist in and interact with this material world.

A material world with which we are free to interact without risking death is impossible. God could no more make a world with which we can freely interact without risking death than God could create a rock so heavy God couldn't pick it up. These are logical impossibilities. But what does this have to do with cancer not being evil?

I see cancer as a messy, ugly, yet necessary byproduct of the ever-changing planet we inhabit. Our world changes continually, and survival for all living things depends on constant adaptation. It is fortunate that all life has the capacity to change. Without that ability, life on this earth would have ceased long ago or would at least be in serious jeopardy now as we face the uncertainties of a rapidly changing global climate. That the blueprints for life—that is, DNA—can and do change, and rather often, makes me immensely grateful to God for having the audacity to create this universe as God did. Ours is a universe not ruled by an iron fist and a mighty thunderclap but guided by a gentle whisper, a still, small voice.

God could have made a fixed world, a spectacular world, but one in which choice and change are impossible. Of course, many people believe God originally did, and that the genetic mutations that give rise to cancer are a result of sin's corrupting influence. I have to reject this line of thought, for it credits sin, not God's creative imagination and power, with the genetic diversity in our world.

If genetic mutations are a result of "the Fall," then the difference between a red-tailed hawk and a red-shouldered hawk—species that even the staunchest young-earth creationists believe arose through evolutionary processes—is due to sin's creative power, not God's. If genetic mutations are a result of the Fall, then diversity among humans is a mark of sin's influence as well. After all, any physical attributes apart from brown skin, hair, and eyes are due to genetic mutations that occurred after the first humans lived, whoever you believe them to be. I doubt many people truly believe that diversity of any kind is a result of sin. I cannot accept such a view of the world.

God could have made a world wherein God's children cannot try to make things better, or conversely fail and mess things up. Likewise, I think there's a chance God could have made a world with which we cannot interact. It is difficult to imagine such a place, and I am not sure it is even possible to have such a world, though I think God could have found a way. But I thank God for not going that route. I wouldn't want to live in a world with no risk of a tree limb crushing me if it meant I couldn't walk in a forest. I wouldn't want to live in a world without sunburn, without drowning, without death if it meant I could not enjoy a sunny day, paddle in a canoe, or take full part in life in a material world, all of which carry risks of injury and death. I am glad God made the world as God did: a diverse and dynamic world, not a uniform and static one.

Sure, it is thanks to a change in the DNA in some stupid rogue cell of mine that I have cancer. Some might say it is not worth the risk of cancer to live in a world with such wondrous capacity for change. Some would also say it is not worth having a world wherein we are free to choose to hate so that we might also be free to choose to love. I am tempted to think this at times. Were I in charge of creating everything, I may have opted for a fixed creation filled with automatons incapable of doing evil—but therefore unable to do good as well.

Thankfully, God knows better than I do. Instead of merely speaking a fixed creation into existence and being done with it, God made a universe of change where the building blocks of all matter are made of spinning, moving, dynamic parts. Change and movement permeates God's creation on every level, even as God's creative word softly echoes through it all. If I believed in a fixed, unchanging creation, I would have serious, troubling questions about cancer. Why God causes or even allows cancer at all would definitely rattle my belief in a God of love. I would likely harbor a great deal of rage toward God, holding God responsible for my cancer, and my faith would be shaken to its foundations. If there were no change in this world, no ability to evolve, no need for DNA to be able to mutate, there would be no reason for cancer. Fortunately, I have been blessed with exposure to a range of views on God's creative processes and for many years have embraced an understanding of an ever-evolving creation.

I remain grateful to God that the world and universe(s) God made are all the more spectacular for their ability to change and adapt, to exhibit God's continual creative power and skill, and to allow us to work as co-creators with God. If cancer, the product of cell division gone awry, is a necessary result of such a splendid and dynamic world—one we can interact with and enjoy—that is fine with me. Even when my own life is at stake.

Chapter 2

Not Everything Happens for a Reason

The Ronald McDonald House of New York City, or just "the Ronald" as the regulars call it, is truly a second home to me. Christina and I lived there for the better part of my first year of treatment and have returned many times for shorter stays, enjoying larger living quarters than a lot of people in New York City, and without roommates too! I cannot imagine how any of my treatment could have worked without the Ronald. Just five short blocks from Sloan Kettering, the Ronald McDonald House allowed us to stay in New York City during my toughest phases of treatment without going bankrupt trying to pay for hotels. Being able to live in the city for months at a time, rather than traveling back and forth from Corning every week or two was a lot easier on me, especially that first year.

Staying at the Ronald also kept me much more active than I would have been otherwise, since I walked to the hospital and back most days, even if I didn't do anything else. I think I took a taxi between the Ronald and the hospital just once, when I was so sick that they had to postpone my chemo for another day. Staying within walking distance of the hospital proved especially beneficial during the great snowpocalypse of 2015 when a couple inches of snow buried the city, shutting down all public transit options and ending the world as people knew it. I got a fever the night of the snowstorm and enjoyed a peaceful, quiet walk through the light flurries on my way to the hospital. It seemed pretty ridiculous to me at the time, since I grew up in the Midwest with lake-effect snow from Lake Michigan being a regular part of every winter. I hadn't yet realized how quickly a couple of inches of slush can pile up in a city with no extra space for snow-banks. At any rate, it was comforting to be able to walk to the hospital no matter the weather. The Ronald's proximity to Sloan Kettering is just one of its many positive attributes.

I'll always remember the overwhelming relief I felt when I first arrived at the Ronald. After a long day of chemo—my first day of chemo, in fact—I walked to my new home where a pair of friendly, sedentary dogs, a basset hound and a Newfoundland, greeted me. They're regulars there too, along with a few other dogs whose owners volunteer their time to brighten people's days. Christina and I especially appreciated the therapy dogs as we had yet to get our own dog, one more part of life put on hold thanks to cancer.

I took a quick tour of the large, plush, shared living room area, complete with a bunch of couches, a fireplace, and a sizable saltwater fish tank that housed, among other creatures, a puffer fish, some kind of parrot-fish that changed colors, and a moray eel. I always liked that fish tank. Then I went upstairs to the spacious dining area with its adjoining kitchens and an impressive, well-stocked pantry. There I ate the first meal I held down for a couple days, tomato soup and grilled cheese.

We all marveled at how well I felt that evening, but it was just because the new chemo hadn't set in yet and I was sufficiently hydrated for the first time that week from a full day of being hooked up to IVs. I also had a take-home hydration backpack, a wonderful bit of technology that allows people who need IV hydration not to be tied down to a clunky IV pole or stuck in a hospital. That was our first exposure to a theme that emerged throughout my treatment: hydration is critical. It affects dozens of other issues and on its own can be the difference between feeling all right and feeling like death is stalking you. Hydration is also difficult. I sometimes needed four liters a day, which is a lot. Keeping me hydrated was a constant struggle throughout my many rounds of chemotherapy, and it played a significant part in several other phases of treatment too.

After that first supper at the Ronald, I finally reached our room, furnished with two single beds, a couch, a desk and chair, a dresser, a TV, and, most important, a bathroom.

I've developed a love/hate relationship with bathrooms over the course of the last few years. Undergoing various types of chemo with equally various side effects ranging from constipation to diarrhea—sometimes manifesting at the same time, a condition I previously would have thought impossible—meant I spent a lot of time in the bathroom. I got to know where public restrooms are in New York City, which is mostly Starbucks, larger parks, and the more concentrated shopping centers like Chelsea Market or Rockefeller Plaza's underground labyrinth. Most sit-down restaurants have bathrooms too, but you can't just waltz in, take care of business, and leave. To be fair, the restrooms at Starbucks are also for customers only, but I count them as public restrooms since my wife and I never minded an excuse to get a latte or Frappuccino or whatever other names those delicious drinks with two days' worth of sugar are called. At the Ronald, I was grateful for my own private bathroom.

Our first room at the Ronald was better than I could have imagined. It even had a nice view overlooking an outdoor courtyard area that was well used in the summertime, especially for dinner. That's another great part of staying at the Ronald. Almost every evening, a group of volunteers comes in and provides supper. Sometimes it's a home-cooked meal made by the volunteers in the kitchens, and sometimes it comes from a nearby restaurant. For patients and I think even more so for caregivers, that's a huge blessing. Food isn't exactly cheap in New York City. Nothing is. That's why the Ronald McDonald House is so important. For people like me and the many families staying there, there is no other option. There is no other place to stay that is remotely affordable and works with nearby hospitals to arrange lodging and take care of as much as possible for guests.

Christina and I settled in and made the Ronald our new home for a while. I won an Xbox One in a drawing held by the NFL when people from their main offices came to serve supper and hand out prizes. I'd never owned any video games before and never would have without cancer. But the escape that they provide has made a lot of rough days go by much quicker. If Einstein hadn't figured out that time is relative, then any gamer would have discovered it by now. Just ten or fifteen minutes of Minecraft makes an hour or two go by in the real world, and I can happily play Star Wars Battlefront for a short break from whatever I'm doing only to find that the sun has set and I've missed a meal. That might not be ideal every day, but on the really rough days when the absolute misery of chemo settles in, it's great. I think everyone going through cancer treatment should have access to video games, and I'm truly curious to see the ways virtual and augmented reality technology becomes integrated with medical care and the role it will play in helping patients cope with difficult realities and the drudgery of unpleasant treatments.

With its many amenities and comforts, the Ronald McDonald House has helped us feel at home and settle into a routine during cancer treatment, and it remains a bright spot in a dark couple of years. The early chemo was terrible, but I expected that. I expected to feel horrible, not to be able to eat or drink much, not to feel like walking or doing anything. I expected to be a cancer patient.

That's because I never struggled to accept my diagnosis of desmoplastic small round cell tumors. The information we had at first was limited, at times self-contradictory, and often just wrong, as we found out while talking to the oncologists at Sloan Kettering. But by any reckoning, the odds were bleak and the treatment would have to be as aggressive as the cancer itself; it has a particularly nasty habit of coming back again and again. But I reasoned that if I had beaten the odds by getting cancer in the first place, I could beat them again. I know that isn't how statistics or probability works, but it seemed better than any other ways of thinking about it. I had no trouble accepting that this was my new life. If anything, I accepted it too well at first.

When it became apparent that my treatments would be a full-time job for a while, I easily adjusted to the idea of life as a cancer patient. I resigned myself to my fate without much of a fuss, telling myself I was being practical, not pessimistic, when I figured I would never ski or snowboard again, never again play hockey or ultimate Frisbee, never again go hiking or canoeing or participate in any of the activities I enjoy. In fact, I started to think of myself first and foremost as a *Cancer Patient*, with all the limitations I thought came inherently with such a title. Cancer patients don't go out to eat. Cancer patients don't go to Broadway plays. Cancer patients don't go to museums. They don't attend sporting events—much less participate in sports. They don't visit parks, they don't go to concerts, they don't really do anything. They sit around sick and tired all the time, barely able to eat, barely able to do more than watch TV in a haze of medications and nausea. A combination of ignorance and laziness—and, to be fair, a really rough time on the first regimen of chemo—threatened to keep me in bed, unable to enjoy life to the fullest.

But DSRCT is classified as a pediatric cancer, and that in some ways has saved my life, or at least saved my life as I know it. Having a pediatric cancer, even though I'm twenty-some years old, qualifies me for housing at the Ronald and means my medical care mostly happens on the pediatric floor at Sloan Kettering.

That means I have spent a great deal of time around dozens of very young people also going through cancer treatment. Something about seeing kids twenty years my junior going through the same slog of treatment has made it impossible to be ungrateful for the comparably long life I have already enjoyed. I learned early in my treatment not to waste time feeling sorry for myself. There's always someone else going through something much worse who would be happy with my situation. Compared to some of the people at Sloan Kettering and the Ronald, I have it pretty easy.

For one thing, I have health insurance. At diagnosis, I had good health insurance through my father's workplace since I was still considered young enough, which meant it didn't matter that cancer treatment had become my full-time job and my wife and I were unemployed. We were both able to quit work and focus on one thing: getting me the treatment I needed. We know plenty of other people who had to continue working to keep their health insurance during a spouse's or child's treatment. Though we're starting to encounter this issue now that we're a little older, I cannot imagine how difficult it would have been for my wife to stay at home working and be unable to spend time with me as I struggled through chemotherapy, radiation, surgery, and more. It would have been immeasurably hard for both of us. There are a lot of people much tougher than we are!

We also didn't have to travel halfway around the world for my treatment. My parents live just a four-hour drive away from New York City in Corning, a lovely small town in Upstate New York. Realistically, it's more like six or eight hours with traffic, but that's still not too bad. To make matters much easier, a couple months into treatment we discovered the Corporate Angel Network, a wonderful program that allows cancer patients to fly for free with one caregiver on corporate jets with extra seats. This means my wife and I can fly for free from the airport just fifteen minutes away from my parents' home and be in New York City in a couple hours via a half-hour flight to New Jersey and a shockingly long shuttle bus ride from New Jersey into the city. Compared to the plight of many people we met at Sloan Kettering and the Ronald McDonald House, we had it easy regarding transportation.

People come to New York City from all across the globe seeking the best possible medical treatment. At times, it seemed most people staying at the Ronald had come from somewhere outside this country, and I found myself wishing I knew more languages than English and some passable Spanish. At the Ronald, we encountered people whose dress, language, and religion brought a wondrous bouquet of variety to what was an otherwise bleak situation. We shared meals, a communal living room, and a hospital with dozens of families who were going through much the same difficulties as us, with the added challenges of navigating cultural and linguistic barriers. All of us, no matter our country of origin, race, religion, or any other part of our identities, stood united in a single desire: to have whoever in our family was sick become healthy again.

That instilled an important lesson in me. We are all simply people—all of us very much the same in the ways that actually matter, regardless of how many differences we might appear to have. Furthermore, the whole of humanity is in fact made stronger by diversity when we unite for common causes. It's an idea that has stuck with me the last few years as divisive, hate-filled rhetoric has gained increasingly solid public footing here in the United States. This is far too important a subject to mention only in passing, so I'll dedicate a sizable chunk of chapter 7 to it, but it also plays too big a role in my experiences at the Ronald not to mention here as well. The essence of the Ronald is family. Everyone who stays there, for however brief a time, gains membership into a wonderful, compassionate, tough group of the loveliest, most courageous people on this earth.

I barely remember my first day of chemotherapy at Sloan Kettering, though I do hold some clear first impressions of the pediatric day hospital, and those proved true with time. I recall being grateful to receive my treatment on a floor full of colors other than beige, with a glass roof overhead allowing views of clouds and birds. It was a far less drab atmosphere than what is found in your average adult hospital unit. I appreciated spending my days in a hospital area filled with music, toys, and a little more life and energy than you usually find in a hospital, even if roving clowns routinely made rounds, cheering up younger kids while I closed my eyes and pretended to be asleep so they'd leave me alone. I didn't want to see any magic tricks or get a balloon animal. I wanted to be left alone, to do nothing, to be a sedentary cancer patient, since that was all I or anyone going through cancer treatment was. Or so I thought.

But I started to look around me and find that it was simply not true. Children with just as much cancer as I had didn't seem to know the rules about being a cancer patient. I saw kids going for rides on their IV poles, playing tag, making art, and shrieking with delight at the simple things in life. It seemed to me that somehow, incredibly, it barely mattered to them that they had cancer. I know that isn't accurate, but it seemed like it—at least on their good days when they felt all right. These kids were hooked up to hydration backpacks like I was, and sometimes had even more going on than I did, like feeding tubes snaking down their noses, something I've never needed. I remember thinking that if only I was young enough not to fully understand the gravity of the situation like those kids, then things might be different. Then I could live life and do what I want. But alas, I knew better, and I made my peace with what I figured my new life would involve.

I stayed in my room and watched a lot of *Top Gear* that first month. Every episode on Netflix, in fact. Then I met a great guy about my age whose college plans took a backseat to osteosarcoma. A state championship-winning basketball player in high school, he told me casually about going to various games at Madison Square Garden on the same day as his chemo. Okay. Message received. Movies might (almost) show cancer only in two forms—as the untreatable killer that leaves its victims too weak to move before killing them, or as the obstacle caught early and overcome by the "fighter" character—but this needn't be the case, even for those who understand their situation exactly. It's entirely possible to have cancer that wasn't caught early, to have little chance of beating it, and to still fully enjoy the best that life has to offer while you can.

So Christina and I started to do more whenever I felt up to it. Our first few weeks in New York City run together in my mind—a rush of new places, unfamiliar faces, and a constant struggle just to get through each day. It's laughable how little we knew about the city when we first got there, and now, having lived there the better part of a year and a half, I cringe to think of the clueless tourist moves we pulled our first month or two in Manhattan. We hadn't gotten the memo about NYC's official winter apparel color (black), and our colorful ski jackets marked us as outsiders. We hailed cabs that didn't have their roof lights on, didn't know what (not who) Duane Reade was or who Billy Joel was, and thought Times Square was someplace worth going. (It isn't. It really isn't. Seriously, stay away. Don't go.)

In the spirit of making the most of the time we had, we said yes to pretty much every free ticket offered to us through the Ronald McDonald House. That's yet another awesome part of staying there: people in New York City who buy tickets to events and then can't attend can donate them to guests of the Ronald. I'm sure some people buy tickets just to donate them because we were offered tickets fairly often.

Through this ticket program, Christina and I were able to attend our first NFL game. Neither team had a chance of making the playoffs, and it was one of the last games of the season, so the outcome didn't matter all that much, but it was still a neat experience. The most appreciated free tickets we received took us to five or six Rangers hockey games, including a playoff game that went into overtime. Like all good citizens of Canada—I have Canadian citizenship through my dad, US through my mom—I love hockey. While Christina isn't into watching hockey or any other televised sports, she does enjoy hockey live. It's hard not to when you get excellent seats for free. We became pretty big Rangers fans.

Seeing the musical *The Lion King* on Broadway impressed us both as well. I may have crossed a line, going despite my blood counts being too low to be in a crowd of people, but I still think it was worth it. I'd do it again without hesitating.

Then I learned the hard way who Billy Joel was. We were offered a pair of tickets that my mom said we had to accept. I declined to go, partly because I didn't know Billy Joel by name, partly because I legitimately felt horrible, and partly because I felt lazy and just wanted to play Minecraft. I hadn't quite learned my lesson yet and still acted like being a cancer patient prevented me from being anything else. I still do sometimes, to be honest. Anyway, my mom and wife went to the concert without me and found themselves seated right across the aisle from George Lucas. They got a picture of the back of his head as proof. Star Wars fanboy that I am, I vowed never again to turn down Billy Joel tickets. Also, now I know who Billy Joel is, and since I knew a bunch of his songs already and hadn't associated his name with them, I'd happily go to a concert of his for its own sake. The point is that I realized that simply accepting my diagnosis was tangential to giving up. We've since found hundreds of ways to make the most of the craziness that is my life, balancing acceptance of my limitations with a desire to do and live as much as possible.

As my understanding of what it means to be a cancer patient evolved, one idea has remained unchanged and was actually reinforced by the young patients around me. Stated simply, it is this: *not everything happens for a reason.*

It's an almost universal trait among humans to try to find meaning amid suffering. And it's fine to wonder why. It's something I'm actively doing in this book. Searching for some meaning or reason for our hardships is a normal part of the human condition. But it's also fraught with peril and has led to what I believe are destructive theologies.

It's impossible to refute the idea that everything happens for a reason without addressing the notion that people who experience suffering are morally culpable for their hardships, so I'll tackle that first. This notion is shockingly prevalent among Christians today, despite being explicitly rejected by Jesus. I think I see or hear some variant of this argument at least weekly as healthcare remains a major issue of contention in the United

States, and each time it pisses me off just a little bit more. This frightful notion manifests itself in all sorts of hideous ways.

I've heard arguments that people who "lead good lives" don't experience health issues. I've seen statements declaring that people with health issues are simply getting what they deserve, reaping the fruits of their choice not to care for their bodies properly. A small part of me is glad such statements are being made. It shows that many people have never personally encountered significant health issues and, as such, are able to remain woefully ignorant of how human health actually works. To an extent, that's the way it should be. I'd rather some people hold to this belief than have everyone agree with me simply because they too have suffered serious illness through no fault of their own. But I'd also enjoy seeing this idea fade into the doleful memories of a less-enlightened past, so I'll present my own arguments against it here.

First, from a scientific and medical perspective, one's health has nothing to do with whether or not one has "led a good life." Sometimes illnesses just happen. This is simply a fact of life. My cancer has no known risk factors. It's just a random glitch, an accidental chromosomal translocation that I don't fully understand. The only thing I've ever done to put myself at a greater-than-normal risk for cancer is receive cancer treatments like radiation. That doesn't mean that, should I develop a secondary cancer down the road, I did the wrong thing by seeking treatment.

Perhaps you think I *am* morally responsible for my cancer. I was diagnosed at age twenty-three after all, and I certainly didn't live a morally perfect life those twenty-three years. Did I do something before I got cancer that doomed me? After all, over the course of my life I've gone seven-for-seven with the "deadly sins." I'm hardly a perfect example to refute the idea that sickness is punishment for wrongdoing.

But what about the babies and children I know at my hospital in New York City? These kids got cancer at young ages. Some were even born with cancer. Can we really blame them for their illness? I struggle to think of a moral failing anyone could commit before being born that would merit their getting cancer as a wake-up call or punishment for their behavior. And that's one of the key problems with this idea. If health and illness are handed out according to some moral point-keeping system, it's being done inconsistently. Cancerous infants aside, we can all think of wonderful people who come down with serious illnesses, just as we can think of some not-so-wonderful people who live exceedingly long, healthy lives. Perhaps if everyone who ascribed to a certain religious or moral code were immune to illness, this idea might be valid. But as it is, this notion ignores the way the world actually works.

I will concede that our life choices can influence our health to an extent. Sometimes lifestyle choices can affect our health status, though certainly not everyone who drinks heavily is equally likely to develop liver problems, not everyone who smokes is equally likely to get lung cancer, and not everyone who exercises regularly is equally protected against a heart attack. Nevertheless, it can be true that our decisions and lifestyles play a role in determining our health, along with a host of other factors outside of our control. But even when someone's actions have negatively influenced their health, dozens of other variables are in play. It isn't fair to blame someone living in a food desert for not eating more fresh produce, for example. It's impossible to know all the reasons someone might be unable to make the healthiest choices during their life, and to hold people morally accountable for the way they were raised or the environment into which they were born is neither fair nor responsible.

Since the simple realities of this world don't seem to be enough to keep some people from blaming those who are ill for getting sick, though, I'll switch tacks. The idea that people who develop health issues somehow brought it upon themselves is refuted several times in the Bible.

I'll start with Job. As I read it, Job can be summarized in two words: "Shit happens." Anything can happen to anyone. The wicked aren't necessarily punished and the righteous aren't always rewarded. Sometimes—most of the time, in fact—life makes little sense from such a perspective.

Job's friends, like many of us today, don't seem to understand this. His three friends are less than helpful in their attempts to rationalize and explain Job's suffering. Rather than assist their friend, they in fact add to his misery as Job is forced to defend himself against their attacks and their unhelpful claims that he has somehow brought disaster upon himself. We learn, however, that what afflicts Job is not some divine retribution for misdeeds, nor is it all part of a painful lesson that God decided Job had to learn in the hardest way possible. It simply happened.

One of Job's friends, some sanctimonious guy named Bildad, says, "If you will seek God and make supplication to the Almighty, if you are pure and upright, surely then he will rouse himself for you and restore to you your rightful place" (8:5-6). To which Job responds, "Indeed I know that this is so; but how can a mortal be just before God?" (9:2). Job further laments as he ponders, "Why do the wicked live on, reach old age, and grow mighty in power?" (21:7). As I understand it, the book of Job spends as much time examining the question, "Why do good things happen to bad people?" as it spends on the question most of us associate with the book, "Why do bad things happen to good people?" In addition, it asserts simultaneously that not only are none righteous before God but also that Job has done nothing to earn his hardships. More to my point, we see that Job does not deserve to suffer hardships through some moral failing on his part, yet there he sits, dejected and in a pile of ashes, scraping at painful sores with a potshard, his health, wealth, and children taken from him. Job has not sinned egregiously, not more than his friends, nor have his friends been more righteous than him. Still, he is afflicted and they are not.

Job's eventual response to this contradiction is to conclude that God must be unjust, and indeed this response may be the only logical one for someone who believes in a morality-based, reward-and-punishment system in which they have committed no particular wrong but endure hardships anyway. I have seen many people who believe hardships are the result of moral failings fall into anger and rage at God when life takes unpleasant turns through no fault of their own. It breaks my heart every time.

I think it breaks God's heart, too, because at this point in the story of Job, God shows up. God does not reveal to Job the reason for his suffering. God does not explain how justice works. God simply challenges Job, reminding Job of his smallness and insignificance compared to God and all God's works. Job subsequently repents of calling God unjust, his only mistake in this whole affair. God then directly rebukes Job's three friends, declaring that "you have not spoken of me what is right, as my servant Job has" (42:7). Ultimately, it is Job, who maintained that he did nothing to bring his difficulties upon himself, who is declared right, and his friends, who sought to blame Job for his own misfortune, who are denounced.

Life isn't quite that cut and dry, and a significant part of why I love Job is the same as why I used to hate it: every time I read Job, I experience both wondrous clarity and profound confusion. And I think that's sort of the point. Job provides some answers, but it also reminds us of how little we can fully understand. It tells us *why not*, but it gives no satisfying answer to *why*. Job highlights that God's purposes and designs are, ultimately, beyond our reckoning. No matter what answers we invent to life's toughest questions, we are unable to truly understand except when God grants us wisdom. Things just happen, and we make fools of ourselves when we declare the reasons they occur.

John 9:1-3 provides another, less-confusing rebuttal of the destructive thinking that blames the ill for their illnesses. This passage tells of Jesus and his disciples encountering a man who was blind from birth. The disciples ask, "Who sinned, this man or his parents, that he was born blind?" Jesus refutes their thinking, answering, "It was not that this man sinned, or his parents, but that the works of God might be displayed in him." Like Job, this doesn't give us a particularly clear or satisfying answer as to *why*, but it clearly shows us *why not*. Ailments and difficulties are not retribution for sin, either ours or our ancestors'. Children born with cancer are not suffering the punishment for their parents' sins. They simply got cancer, just like the man in John was blind through no moral failing of his or of anyone else's.

This ties back into what I said in the previous chapter about rain and sunshine: it doesn't matter if we are righteous or not; we will experience all kinds of weather either way. Another lesson we can take from that passage is not to assume that anyone's circumstances arise from their moral failings and successes. First, we cannot actually say whether any circumstances are good or bad to begin with. Staying with the example of rain and sunshine, we need both in balance. We might prefer one or hate the other, but we still need both. They aren't good and they aren't evil. If we cannot know whether someone's circumstances are good or evil, then how much less should we point to someone's right or wrong actions as the cause of the circumstances? As nice as it would be to have a personal weather system rewarding us for our good behavior and punishing us—or perhaps just others—for wrong-doings, that isn't how it works here on earth. The systems of this world do not consider the morals of the people they affect; they simply operate more or less as God created them to operate. We could argue about the extent to which the systems of the world function exactly as God made them compared to the ways sin has potentially corrupted them, but this book isn't the place for that. Ultimately, these systems work without considering the moral behavior of those they affect.

As I said before, cancer and weather are not evil. They can and do cause suffering, and the suffering they cause is indeed evil, but I don't believe they're evil on their own. I think they just *are*. As I see it, to say that people bring morally neutral circumstances upon themselves through their misdeeds is logically incoherent.

Related closely to this is the truly frightful notion that God inflicts unpleasantness upon those who need to learn valuable life lessons. Thankfully, I never put any stock into that idea, or I could worry myself to death wondering what I should be learning and hoping that I have learned it well enough to leave the past three years in the past. Under such a schema, I would view any future relapse of cancer as my fault for not *really* learning whatever it was God was trying to teach me.

Not only would that be unhealthy and unhelpful for my mental state, but it would also lead me to a warped view of God or, more accurately and much worse, to a view of a warped God. A God who doles out cancer and other hardships just so we may learn something about the nature of life flies in the face of everything I understand about God. It goes against logic and reason, against my own relationship with God, and against any of Jesus' teachings that I know. Sure, there are plenty of times when the Bible depicts God as smiting people in various ways for this or that, but Jesus never says anything to support such ideas and in fact actively refutes them. I think such stories simply reflect the culture and worldviews of the biblical authors who wrote those accounts and shouldn't be given more credence than Jesus, the fullest and clearest revelation of God we have. And we should remember that even the accounts of him that we have are colored by the authors' biases and the cultural rift between the ancient Near East and here and now.

If God were to hand out hardships for the sake of personal growth, then we would be right to grumble about who gets how much. We all know people who could use a little affliction for the sake of learning an important lesson, yet some people just never seem to have anything serious go wrong in their lives. Perhaps God only cares about some people, then, and cares so much about them that God smites them with difficulties due to some weird brand of tough love. As Tevye laments in *Fiddler on the Roof,* "We are your chosen people. But, once in a while, can't you choose someone else?" Such a view can easily lead to the feeling that God is picking on us and perhaps just doesn't care about people living comparably easy lives.

As someone who believes that the redemptive work of Jesus was done for all humanity, though, I find this idea vastly troubling. Since Jesus came to expand God's message of love to all people, no matter who or what they may be, it seems unfair of God to bless some of us with hardships that make us better while letting others coast by in their immaturity. This, to me, is not unlike how unfair it would be if God made some people with heaven in mind while creating others merely to be fodder for the flames of hell.

This leads me to my next point. People don't necessarily need hardships to grow. Plenty of great thinkers and mature, wonderful people have gotten by without cancer, famines, extreme poverty, or other afflictions, and have still been decent, selfless people who strove to do good for others. If you believe God causes hardships so that we may grow, the obvious question to ask is, "Couldn't you have taught me this an easier way?" And the answer is almost always yes. I didn't absolutely need cancer to learn what I have learned these past few years. I do think I have learned much more, and far more quickly, than I might have otherwise. But one does not need to be so blatantly confronted with one's mortality to gain a better perspective on life. Could a 20 percent chance of living five years after diagnosis have taught me the same lessons equally as well as my 15 percent chance? Probably.

The darker side of the coin is that hardships do not always help people grow or mature. Plenty of people break under the strain of difficulties. It's easy to begin a downward spiral of increasingly despairing thoughts, becoming able only to ask, "Why me?" when you receive yet another piece of bad news. And I certainly do not mean to blame anyone for feeling this way. Sometimes life really is hard and seems impossible. I remember thinking during the first few days of my treatment that this wasn't worth going through if it didn't actually prolong my life, and if progress didn't happen soon I figured I'd think about starting palliative care rather than continuing to fight my cancer. I get it. Life sucks sometimes. Sometimes we can't help wondering why we must endure the hardships before us. I just don't find it logically coherent or helpful to answer such questions with an explanation about a need for personal growth that can only be achieved through difficulty.

I will concede something here. The God I know and love has taught me many things through my trials of the past three-plus years. If that weren't true, I wouldn't have bothered writing this book. Each chapter contains lessons I've learned—am still learning—during my experiences with cancer treatments. In fact, many of these life lessons could not have been taught more effectively than they were through my difficulties. So can God use hardships like cancer to teach people lessons, to help them grow? Absolutely. No matter how dire our circumstances may seem, they are never beyond God's capacity to work good in this world. Did I need cancer to understand the lessons I have learned this past year? Sort of, yeah. At least, I learned them more quickly and intensely than I might have otherwise. But could I have lived happily and still matured and grown without learning these lessons the way I did? Yes, definitely. I hope the beautiful balance here is clear. God by no means causes our afflictions so that we might grow; rather, through our afflictions God grows us.

Chapter 3

I Should Be Dead Already

Somehow I made it through those first few rounds of debilitating chemotherapy. It felt much longer than the month and a half or so that it lasted, and I never looked back—at least not until now as I write about it. I simply grit my teeth for what came next: the real chemo, the tough chemo, the chemo that would take my hair and send my blood counts plummeting, and maybe, just maybe, have some effect on the tumors inside me. But before I could start that, I had a safety net to set up.

At Sloan Kettering, it's common practice to harvest stem cells from patients before they begin chemotherapy regimens that are likely to lower their blood counts dramatically. Those stem cells can be given back to the patients later to boost their immune system after the most intense treatment ends. Harvesting stem cells is doubtless a far more difficult and involved process than I'm aware of, but for me it was pretty straightforward.

I got a shot every morning for a few days to stimulate my bone marrow, and then I had to sit still for a couple of hours without moving my left arm while I watched a movie on my iPad. It grows progressively more difficult to hold your arm still when you have to, but the giant metal needle in the crook of my elbow made it a little easier, since I didn't think it would feel so great to try moving while it was stuck in me. My blood drained from my left arm, went through a tube into a sizable machine that, if I remember correctly, used a centrifuge to separate the stem cells from the rest of my blood. Then my blood—sans stem cells—returned to me, the tube coiling around a heating element first so that it entered my right arm at body temperature. It only took me one try to get several times the stem cell count they wanted, and I was grateful for that. Reportedly, it can take three or four days of harvesting to get enough stem cells, so I got off easy in that regard. Then, with my stem cells collected, it was time to start the real chemo.

I can't remember exactly when I started the first of several tougher chemotherapy cycles, or even the names of all the different drugs I received. Cyclophosphamide is the only one I know off the top of my head, and that's just because I took it in pill form as part of a different course of treatment for more than a year. With the new regimen of chemo came a change in side effects. I didn't feel quite as violently sick, and I didn't have any more complications like C. diff messing everything up. I did experience the overall sense of malaise that I call "feeling chemo-y." It's not terrible, or at least not the worst thing ever, but it is all encompassing and feels undeniably not right. I suppose that's the best way to describe it. Rather than the sensation that something particular is wrong, "feeling chemo-y" is the pervasive sense that everything is just not right. In a lot of ways, that's worse. I felt physically exhausted, though my mind was about as alert as could be expected. An overarching sensation of something being amiss, toxic, and unbalanced sat in my torso. I didn't have heartburn exactly, but something like heartburn's obnoxious, nauseating cousin constantly lurked in my chest. If "feeling chemo-y" had a color, it would be yellow. Not a nice yellow but a sickly, infected yellow.

Eating became a battle. I felt hungry and grotesquely full at the same time, craved food and despised it in one roiling circle of ever-changing sensations. I'd ask for food regularly enough, but often by the time it arrived the smell of it would make me feel the impending rush of vomit. I learned eventually to eat more and head it off, for in part what I felt was just hunger, processed differently than I was used to. If I could stay ahead of it, everything went far smoother. But I often fell behind and struggled to eat enough to feel like eating at all.

It was still far easier than my first three cycles of chemo, those low-dose drugs from an experimental protocol that at times caused abdominal pain so bad I could scarcely move, at least not without swearing more than seemed appropriate for a pediatric hospital.

Some days I needed two infusions of a bolus, a giant bag of IV hydration, before I could start the new, higher-dose chemo. Some days I came to the hospital by 7 AM and didn't leave until 8 PM. I napped when I could, finished watching all of *Top Gear* on Netflix, and got into the habit of writing more. I finished writing the Tamyth Trilogy, my young adult fantasy series, while on the most intense cycles of chemo. I wrote at a feverish pace whenever I had time and felt lucid enough not to turn the series into something Lewis Carroll might have written. With my first major surgery looming, I wanted to finish the series—which I began when I was fourteen and restarted in college—as soon as possible.

I didn't exactly expect to die in surgery, but I didn't really think I'd live either. At least, not for very long, whether I died from surgery specifically or from cancer more generally. I don't think I was overly morbid about it. The simple fact was that, in all likelihood, I didn't have a lot longer to live, so I decided to be completely fine with the prospect of dying, even as I hoped I'd live long enough to accomplish some of my goals. I knew I would regret not finishing the Tamyth Trilogy, just like now, as I write this, I know I'll feel profoundly dissatisfied if I don't finish this book or the others I'm currently writing.

These intense cycles of chemotherapy lasted three weeks. The first week, I received infusions of chemo for two or three days, then I continued going to the hospital for IV hydration. After that, I had two weeks off to recover. I liked those two weeks off. Usually by the second off-week I'd be feeling well enough to do more than sit around all day. We managed to explore more of New York City during the recovery weeks. Some of my favorite sites include the American Museum of Natural History, the Met, the New York Public Library with adjacent Bryant Park, and a secret spot in Central Park on a pleasant little knoll with a lovely view of some stately trees. That Central Park spot is one of my favorite places to sit and read. I once saw a man walking his pet tortoise there, which provides a good indication of the relaxed pace and quiet tranquility of this undisclosed locale. There's also a bathroom close by, so it's perfect for me.

My wife and I happily accepted more Rangers tickets during this time, and later, in the spring, we went to the Bronx Zoo on a trip organized by the Ronald McDonald House. I had just finished a cycle of chemo the day before, so we had to disconnect my hydration backpack ourselves on the bus before we went into the zoo. It was totally worth it. My second-favorite zoo (Smithsonian Zoo in D.C. will always be number one), the Bronx Zoo definitely puts the "park" in "zoological park." It feels enormous, and you can walk a long way between exhibits, almost forgetting you're touring a zoo and not just strolling through a beautiful city park or even a stretch of quiet countryside.

On the whole, the higher-dose chemotherapy went well. It also reinforced a mantra that many of the doctors repeated again and again: chemo affects everyone differently. I had such a rough time on the low-dose, generally tolerable chemo that at first I could scarcely imagine moving to higher doses of tougher chemotherapy drugs that tended to give people a harder time. If I was throwing up most days on the easy stuff, surely I'd be sick constantly on the harder drugs. But that proved wrong, and overall the treatment plan progressed smoothly.

"Overall" is the key word. I made a couple feverish late-night trips to the inpatient center, sometimes staying a week or more until my blood counts rose sufficiently during my recovery periods. As my blood counts dropped with each cycle of chemo, I grew increasingly light-headed and fatigued, and a few times I needed transfusions.

Sometimes my platelets were low, but my hemoglobin levels, among others, were doing well enough so that I only needed platelet transfusions. Those were fun because, as we discovered around 2 a.m. one night, I'm allergic to platelet transfusions, most likely because of the additives and preservatives that keep platelet samples stable and viable before they're infused. I woke up with one eye swollen shut and a terrible itching all over. Thankfully none of the swelling went to my throat, but it was still unsettling since it took a while for the Benadryl and other drugs they gave me to kick in. They triple pre-medicated me before platelet transfusions from that point on.

My blood counts also affected what I was and was not supposed to eat. I've already talked about some of the battles I had with food during this time, but one other difficulty came into play with this new chemotherapy regimen. Since my blood counts started dropping during each cycle of treatment and my immune system grew suppressed, I was forced to follow a low-microbial diet, which means I couldn't eat any fresh fruits or vegetables. Instead, I had to eat more delicious, processed foods, like anything from a can. It was so rough. I joke about it, but it was actually tough, much more so on Christina I think than it was on me. She kept track far better than I did of what seemingly random foods I could or couldn't eat. I was allowed some but not all cheese, and I could eat any kind of bread but challah bread—because of the eggs, I guess. Christina certainly outdid herself as a chef, and I can't imagine the frustrations of making food to fit dietary guidelines for someone as finicky as I was at the time.

Hiccups also made these rounds of chemo interesting. These weren't your average, run-of-the-mill hiccups. They were, if I may say so myself, impressively loud and very annoying. I got a pill to help with them, and that usually made them go away. The hiccups certainly weren't the worst side effect of any of my treatment, but they remain one of the weirdest.

I slogged and skipped my way through a few rounds of chemotherapy, at times exhausted to my core by the fourteen-hour days at the hospital, at other times enjoying some of the best sights and activities New York City has to offer.

Then came the first real surgery.

Scheduled to last somewhere between six and fourteen hours, my first tumor resection surgery would mark the beginning of actually getting the cancer removed. Chemotherapy might be able to slow the growth of my tumors, or perhaps even keep the disease stable, but it was never expected to shrink my tumors, much less get rid of them. No amount of chemo would ever take care of the several pounds of tumor burden in my body. Only surgery could remove them.

So, in preparation for spending most of a day under anesthesia, I mixed a whole bottle of Miralax into two liters of ginger ale and drank all of it the night before to clear my system. Given my previous difficulty with nausea and anesthesia, I got a scopolamine patch before I went to the operating room and had a bunch of Zofran infused while I was under. I woke up about seven or eight hours later in the recovery room, feeling remarkably all right, thanks to my epidural. My only real complaint was the naso-gastric (NG) tube that ran down my nose and throat to vacuum out my stomach, which remained necessary for several days, as it took a while for my insides to wake up and start running in the proper direction again. The NG tube remains my least favorite part of major surgeries, since it dried out my throat terribly. My second least-favorite part of recovering from major surgery is having a Foley catheter. Foley catheters are nice in a way, since the last thing I want to do when I have a fresh incision from my sternum to my pelvis is get up and walk every time I need to pee, but mostly they're annoying, uncomfortable, and stupid.

I'd still take surgery over chemo any day, though. Out of all the treatments I've had over the last few years, surgery makes the most sense to me. With surgery, I wake up and see what I need to deal with, and I make myself get up and walk and recover as soon as possible. Surgery leaves visible, easily understandable wounds that heal pretty quickly, in my experience. By comparison, chemo makes me feel terrible and has no visible physical effects aside from hair loss and weak, thin lines in my fingernails. But with surgery it's easy to see what hurts and what needs to heal, and to an extent how quickly I recover from surgery falls under my control. The more I make myself get up and walk around, the easier it becomes to move and the faster I can leave the hospital.

I spent the first night after surgery in the recovery room, where I didn't sleep much, asked for ice chips and water far more often than they were able to give me any, and listened to the staff talk at 4 a.m. about *Game of Thrones* and *Scandal.* I also smelled the smoke from a nearby apartment fire, which was interesting and a touch disconcerting. Most of my major surgery recoveries started with one day in which I felt that I'd never get better, or at least I couldn't imagine recovering, since I felt so profoundly beat up. But the next few days consisted of making myself sit up, get out of bed, walk painfully slowly along the hospital hallway, and start eating Jell-O. I had a chest tube draining excess fluid from my chest, which they took out in the recovery room the first day after surgery. Later, I got my epidural, Foley catheter, and finally my NG tube removed. I pushed myself pretty hard and walked more and more laps of the hallway until, six days later, they cleared me to walk myself out of the hospital and go back to the Ronald McDonald House.

I'm a bit inclined to brag about how short a time it took me to recover from my surgery, and I like to think it's because I'm super cool or tough, but really I just got lucky and was blessed to have everything go well. It wasn't due to anything special about me or anything I did. And that's an important point I want to make: people receiving cancer treatment aren't warriors or fighters. Indeed, cancer isn't a battle at all.

I know that contradicts the way our culture views cancer, but as far as I've experienced this disease, it's absolutely true. Cancer isn't a fight, and we patients aren't necessarily brave. I know the nearly unanimous response when someone is diagnosed with cancer is to call the person "brave" or "courageous," assuring ourselves that our loved one is a fighter who can beat this new affliction. We like to comfort ourselves with reminders that our beloved is a warrior who will kick cancer's butt, even sharing stories of times they've overcome something difficult before.

That's garbage.

It doesn't matter how strong or courageous someone is. That strength, that courage won't cure their cancer. Only treatments like chemotherapy, surgery, and radiation can get rid of someone's cancer. Being brave, stoic, or tough helps people deal with such treatments, sure. But bravery and stoicism aren't a viable treatment in themselves, and they don't guarantee a positive outcome. I know more than a dozen people who would still be alive today if it were.

I understand that cancer is scary and people like to feel as if there's something they can do about it. We don't like things that are beyond our control. It makes us feel better to think that as long as we're brave enough and determined to fight, we'll be okay even if we get cancer. But cancer doesn't know or care. Cancer just *is*. Cancer is a disease, not a battle, and we need to be realistic about that.

Also, not everyone who gets cancer is brave. I don't consider myself brave for getting through more than three years of cancer treatment. I simply haven't died yet. That's it. It's also worth noting that not everyone who gets cancer feels like they can fight it or even wants to fight it. Telling someone they're tough and brave and can beat it when they don't feel that way isn't very helpful. Besides, bravery doesn't always mean a willingness to fight. In a lot of ways, it's braver to accept our own mortality than to do whatever it takes to stay alive simply because we're afraid of death.

For me, it's best not to say that someone is brave, a fighter, or will kick cancer's butt. We can't know that, and it implies that someone who dies might not have been enough of a fighter or had the right kick-butt attitude. When someone gets cancer, let's think about that person, not about platitudes to make ourselves feel better about their situation. Let's just be there for them, whether they're facing it "bravely" or not, whatever that even looks like.

By whatever means, my incision healed splendidly, my insides kicked back into gear in short order, and I didn't have to deal with any untoward setbacks. The first few times I sat up or tried walking were agony, but I can handle a couple days of difficulty when the payoff is seven to eight pounds of tumor removed—along with my appendix, spleen, and something called an omentum that I'd never heard of before and apparently don't particularly need. I thought I might feel lighter, emptier, after the surgery, but there was enough inflammation, irritation, and fluid in my abdomen that I actually felt fuller than before.

On the whole, though, I felt significantly better after surgery. Physically, I was relieved of seven or eight pounds of useless blobs taking up space in my abdomen and making me feel sick all the time. I also had an awesome new foot-long scar running down my stomach, and I now felt like I could handle any surgery or treatment they might throw my way. My confidence that things would work out rose, even as I tempered my expectations with reality and with daily reminders that my life expectancy was not long. In fact, I'd already outlived it.

I should be dead already, but I don't worry about that.

By my reckoning, I should have died sometime in February or March of 2015. At that point, my cancer should have taken hold of my lungs or perhaps caused a kidney to rupture. Of course, I can't say which would have come first or exactly when I would have died without any treatment. But the cancer progressing to my lungs and blocking my kidneys from draining were the doctors' chief concerns at first, so I tend to think that one of those would have done me in had they not been addressed. I remember the exact moment in March when it hit me that, had I been born even thirty years ago and only had access to the care available at the time, I would be dead already.

One day, my wife Christina and I were walking back from Central Park and had only a few blocks to go before we reached our home, the Ronald McDonald House. I'm not sure what prompted my train of thought, but somehow I was imagining living in medieval Europe, and it occurred to me that applying leeches would likely have been the best treatment that anyone then and there could have offered to me. My thoughts quickly turned to the many advances in medical care over the years, and I realized that, as someone who was scheduled to get a Phase I trial of an experimental treatment in a few months, even a year ago my chances might have been worse than they were today. Especially at Sloan Kettering, new ideas and innovative treatments continually emerge. I'm only alive today because of the latest and best medical care in the world.

That level of medical attention has allowed me to pass milestones in my life I all but forgot about and never expected to reach after I started life as a cancer patient. I lived to see my second wedding anniversary, then my third as of the time I began writing this book. Now my fourth and fifth have come around, which highlight how long it takes to find a publisher and also how we never really know what will happen. None of these anniversaries seemed like days I was likely to see, especially when I was first diagnosed. My past three birthdays also snuck up on me. Every year, I'm pleasantly surprised when my birthday rolls around, even as I don't seriously expect to reach the next one. I always gave myself a fifty-fifty chance of going another year, if I had to pick numbers. We'll see.

Events like our birthday—Christina and I were born about twenty minutes apart on the same day—or anniversary have taken on new significance for me. During my first year of treatment, I did not especially look forward to turning twenty-four. Nothing significant happens at that age in our society. Twenty-five, sure. Once I turned twenty-five, I could rent a car in this country without paying a lot of extra money, which has been useful once so far. But there's nothing too special about being twenty-four that I can think of—no significance, milestone, or perk that comes with the age.

I also never quite understood the idea of celebrating a birthday anyway, so it wasn't too hard for me to be okay with the idea of not having another one when I first started cancer treatment and did not expect to live much longer.

Now, I have always loved celebrating my birthday. Presents, attention, parties, cake: it was all fine by me. But I never understood why we do it. I used to think, *It's not like I accomplished anything.* I didn't choose to be born on this particular date, so why celebrate it? But now I understand better. I still don't think I've accomplished all that much in getting to another birthday—the doctors are the ones who should be celebrated—but there is certainly something worth celebrating on a birthday. Birthdays are about celebrating yet another year that someone has been privileged to be alive. Birthdays are about being grateful for the time we have been given with one another. Birthdays are about appreciating the gift of life, marking the slow, steady march of time across our lives, and being glad for every year we get on this planet. They're a chance to celebrate someone and be grateful they've lived as long as they have while hoping for many more years with them. In light of a bleak cancer diagnosis, a birthday seems suddenly worth celebrating.

That brings up one of my pet peeves. Some people dread birthdays and getting older. There are those who lie about their age, complain about going "over the hill," and who see each increase in the numerical value of their age as a curse, not a blessing. Maybe because I'm only twenty-seven it's easy for me to call that foolish, but I get upset when people complain about another year of life they've enjoyed. After all, getting older is the only way to live longer.

So I for one will be happy, not heartbroken, if I ever reach a milestone birthday like my fortieth, or even my next one. I enjoy fewer guarantees that I'll reach my next birthday than most people, and I hope I don't take that for granted again. So far, I've gotten an extra four years of life, and I'm still counting. I should be filled with gratitude every moment that I live, for I truly am living on borrowed time.

Each and every day multiple reminders of my cancer pop up, ranging from my annoyingly frequent need for a bathroom to the sight of my surgical scars and the nausea and fatigue from my continuing chemotherapy. I cannot go long without something imploring me to be more thankful, to take a step back and not take life—both the simple fact that I'm alive and the quality of life that I enjoy—for granted.

But still, hours go by when I forget to appreciate even the most basic blessings, like the fact that I haven't died yet. Whole days pass when my discomfort or nausea is merely an annoyance and the sight of my scars makes me think only of how badass I am now. (If you saw my scars you would agree. They're pretty legit.) Every morning when I wake up, I start another day that I was by no means guaranteed to get. In light of that, at the beginning of this whole ordeal I resolved to make the most of every moment. I also decided that, if I had only a week or two left to live, I'd want them to be fun but I'd also want them to be reasonably normal. It just seems like the logical way to live, especially in my circumstances.

This is also an idea taught by Jesus. I have long valued and fairly easily lived according to the theme of Matthew 6:25-34, which implores us not to worry. Jesus asks, "Can any of you by worrying add a single hour to your span of life?" (6:28). If that weren't enough, the section ends with the imperative, "do not worry about tomorrow, for tomorrow will bring worries of its own. Today's trouble is enough for today" (6:34). I think a big reason this is one of my favorite ideas in the Bible is that it mirrors what I've experienced with cancer. There's enough going on today, this hour, this minute, that it isn't always worth it to think too far ahead. I have to live in the moment, to enjoy the borrowed time I'm on while I have it.

In light of that, I try my best to live like I would without cancer, to refuse to let it ruin my life, cripple me with fear and doubt, or make me do something crazy like forgo treatment and max out my credit card by traveling everywhere I've ever wanted to see in the next month. In my view, this passage means to keep things in perspective, take on smaller, more manageable chunks of worry, and refocus on the present if tomorrow's troubles intrude on today.

To be clear, this passage does not say that those who worry or experience anxiety have less faith than those who don't, and it certainly doesn't justify the too-prevalent idea that those with mental illness should only seek a pastor's counseling instead of therapy with a certified counselor. As little as I worry and as disinclined as I am toward anxiety and depression, I've still needed counseling during my ordeal with cancer, both on my own and with my wife. The idea that people just need more faith, not counseling, for their mental health struggles is part of the same horrid theology that forgoes medical treatment for physical ailments in favor of prayers for healing. (For more on that, see chapter 4.)

The goal of living in the moment has been a bit of a balancing act, and I haven't always performed it perfectly. On one side, I don't want to live ruled by fear or worry that prevents me from enjoying the here and now. But I also want to make sure I don't waste my time and that I make a concerted effort to do the things I know I would regret leaving unfinished. That's why I've invested so much time since my diagnosis in activities like riding roller coasters, traveling, playing disc golf, and skiing and snowboarding. Fun things, maybe silly things, but things I enjoy that I want to do while I can. I've also increased my efforts in more serious areas, like visiting with friends and family and enjoying quality time with my wife. I've invested a lot of time in writing too. Since my cancer diagnosis, I have tried to find balance in a range of activities, from the important things in life to the fun stuff. And mostly it has worked.

But sometimes I fear that in trying to maintain normalcy, I neglect to appreciate life like I should. It is a constant balancing act to live normally while remaining in a state of awe and thankfulness that I am still living. In my experience, though, the most rewarding parts of life are those that require care and balance. Holding a deep appreciation for life in balance with a carefree lifestyle spent enjoying the present moment is difficult. I certainly don't have all the answers of how best to do this, but I am certain that my life has been far richer since I started to make a conscious effort in this area. Sometimes trying is more important than succeeding.

Chapter 4

Prayer Is Weird

Eleven days after my surgery, I had forty-some staples taken out, each one feeling like a mosquito bite as it went. That doesn't seem bad, but it starts to add up after a while. My incision site continued healing well and I began to feel less full inside, though I still had several pounds of tumor left in me. I expected to feel a void where my spleen had been too, but that never happened. I simply felt a little more normal, a little less filled with unnecessary blobs of cells growing purely for the sake of growth. If you look closely at me now, you can see that my stomach is not quite symmetric, and the left side just beneath my ribs sticks out a little less than the right side, but nobody is perfectly symmetric anyways, and I have no idea if that's a result of my splenectomy or if it's related more generally to all the surgeries I've had. The only tangible sign of my missing spleen in the days and months following this surgery was a feeling of pressure in my left shoulder when I ate. I still feel it if I eat too much too quickly, though the frequency and intensity have decreased in the years since this surgery. The human nervous system is a fickle, complex beast, and I guess there's some connection from the spleen to the left shoulder that can cause this sensation. It was hardly the most difficult part of recovering from this surgery, though.

I avoided stairs or taking long strides for a couple weeks, and I had to step gingerly over curbs when walking around New York City. My stomach still felt deeply sore, like I had somehow done a few hundred sit-ups an hour ago and needed to recover. Even so, I healed quickly, and within a month I felt more or less completely recovered.

Chemo resumed two weeks after surgery. I needed some time off to heal fully, since the treatment slows cell growth. My next surgery was scheduled for the end of May, almost two months away, too long to go without some sort of treatment. This was more of the same intense type of chemo, and it proceeded like before. I felt weird and terrible, didn't want to eat for a few days when I got my infusions, and slept a lot. Basically, it was no fun. I didn't have any significant complications, though, and I still had my eyebrows so I didn't look like death or Voldemort or Kermit the Frog, as happened a little later.

By now it was fully spring in NYC, a wonderful time when life bursts forth and everything smells putrid, like the odors of a thousand varieties of discarded refuse are waking up from a long hibernation. Gone were the trash-infused snowbanks, replaced with foul gray water pooling along the curbs. Flowers and leaves lent life, color, and a more pleasant aroma to the streets. It was a vibrant, exciting time to be in the city. Christina and I spent more time in the courtyard at the Ronald, and I ate a lot of ice cream sandwiches. We discovered our favorite spot in Central Park. We explored museums and enjoyed a bit more of what living in the largest city in the country has to offer. It felt increasingly normal and less like life on hold.

Our time at the Ronald and Sloan Kettering became increasingly normal and routine as well. Names attached themselves to more and more of the familiar faces around us. I got to know several doctors, each with their own style, their own way of dealing with their demanding, heart-wrenching line of work. Some approached everything with quiet compassion that belied their fiery determination to fight as hard as possible for the lives of their patients. Other doctors acted as if this were all very normal, which of course for them it was. Some used humor or at least attempted it.

I vividly remember one day in particular, sitting in the exam chair in the office of the head of the pediatric department. He's a wonderful guy, but his jokes are genuinely terrible.

He burst into the room, questions blazing.

"Is your nose running?" he asked urgently.

"A bit, yeah." My nose always ran a little now that all my hair, including my nose hair, was gone.

"Hmm. Do your feet smell?" he said, sounding serious.

"Not more than usual," I replied, confused. Could this be some dangerous sign of something going wrong with my chemo?

"Well, if your nose is running and your feet smell, just tell them to switch places."

I knew then that this doctor must be a father, in spirit at least.

Spring ran into summer, and chemo gave way to more surgery. This time they opened me from sternum to pubic bone and took out another eight pounds of tumor. The procedure lasted about seven hours. They also removed fourteen centimeters of my large intestine, since there was a tumor wrapping tightly around it. This meant I woke up with an ileostomy bag. It had been a strong possibility with my first surgery and was basically a necessity with this second one, so I wasn't surprised, but it was one of the first things I asked about when I woke up.

The ileostomy was a way to reroute my body's solid waste through a hole in the right side of my stomach and into a pouch. I didn't like the ileostomy bag, but I also didn't hate it as much as I thought I might. It at least made recovery easier. I didn't have to get out of bed to use the bathroom, at least not until my Foley catheter came out. Even then, the ileostomy bag meant I could control when I had to "go to the bathroom," that is, simply empty the bag. It filled in three to seven hours, and I never had an urgent feeling of needing to go to the bathroom. I just emptied the bag when it was convenient and never had to worry about rushing to a bathroom.

I also had some complications and hassles with the ileostomy. The bag essentially used a powerful, ring-shaped sticker to stay attached around the opening—officially called a "stoma"—in my body, and that sticker didn't always stick. Sometimes the waste would flow under part of the sticker and slowly start to work it loose. Sometimes I looked down and found a brown wet stain on my t-shirt.

As my hair regrew, given a short break from chemo for this major surgery, I encountered another difficulty of having an ileostomy. The bag has to be changed when the sticker loses its adhesive ability, and each time it became increasingly painful as more and more hair on my stomach pulled out with the bag changes. I did eventually shave my stomach around the area, but we were on a trip to visit family in Wisconsin and Michigan at the time this started, so it didn't happen as quickly as it probably should have.

Sometimes the sticker ring part would repeatedly bubble up and allow the discharge to sit against my skin, which basically gave me diaper rash and led to a more severe breakdown. After a couple months, I constantly dealt with skin breakdown all around the stoma, and it burned more or less continually. I was ready for the ileostomy to go.

But in the years since it was removed, I've found myself at times wishing to have it back. It was nice never having to worry about suddenly needing a bathroom, and it was a lot more convenient to open a spout and empty the bag when it got full than it is to find a bathroom whenever my body says I need one. I dream sometimes about a future wherein technology allows us to transcend the messy details of living in fleshy bodies, and chief among these fantasies are ileostomy bags, or something like them but far more comfortable, easy, and convenient. A spigot, perhaps, one that we need to open only when we wake in the morning and before we go to sleep at night, to eliminate all our bodily wastes.

Ileostomy bag and all, I walked out of the hospital and returned to the Ronald six days after this surgery. It was another surprisingly fast recovery; by the day after the operation, I had moved from Jell-O to mac and cheese with hotdogs, which may seem like an unhealthy food choice, but sometimes the stomach wants what the stomach wants. Or at least the tongue does.

After this surgery, I spent a couple months with the bag and had another two rounds of chemo. Since this chemo regimen consisted of two days of chemo infusions, the rest of the week getting IV hydration, and then two off-weeks, it meant I had some free time to do a little traveling. My whole family went to Wisconsin during this time, in the off-week of chemo. Most of my mother's side of the family lives in the Milwaukee area, and I was a groomsman in my cousin's wedding, so we spent a wonderful few days visiting with everyone there.

From Wisconsin we went on to Michigan, meeting up with Christina's sister and parents to go to her grandparents' home in Oscoda, a tiny, quiet town on Lake Huron. It was a lovely, relaxing time, though by now the stents in my ureters were starting to give me trouble to the point that it hurt to walk or pee. By the time we got home from this trip, I could barely walk without everything burning, and I constantly felt that I had to pee, but when I did it felt even worse. Thankfully, I was already scheduled for another surgery—this time in my chest—and they would remove the stents for me. I no longer needed them since the tumors in my stomach were mostly removed by now, and nothing threatened to pinch off my ureters and back up my kidneys.

This surgery was comparably minor. It was done laparoscopically, which is a fancy way of saying the doctors only needed to make three little holes and use tiny gadgets and a camera to go into my chest. Since I'd had trouble with nausea after previous surgeries, I again used a scopolamine patch, which is like a tiny round bandage that went behind my ear. I put on the patch the afternoon before my surgery, and that evening I noticed a few small, red bumps around it. By the time I woke up from surgery, the bumps had turned itchy and spread more. It seemed that I was allergic to the scopolamine patch. But no allergy treatments worked, and for a day or two it just got worse. Then it became clear that I had shingles.

Shingles suck.

They itch, but they feel far worse than that. They itch your very nerves. They sting, they pinch, they feel like needles, like your nerves are falling asleep and waking up at the same time. The surgery recovery was comparably easy. I was basically back to normal within a couple days. The shingles, though, took a couple of weeks to clear up. Even now, years later, I still feel a twinge every so often on the left side of my head, especially behind my ear—especially when I think about shingles or write about them. (Excuse me a second while I scratch myself.)

After the shingles started clearing, I had a little time off before I started chemo again. Some of my dad's friends from work invited us to their home on one of the Finger Lakes, so we spent a few days there enjoying the view and waterskiing. For my part, I just drove the boat, not feeling up to anything so physically demanding.

Then I did another round of chemo. It went as smoothly as possible, but it still sucked and I don't want to talk about it.

After a week in the hospital for chemo, Christina and I headed up to Lake Placid in the Adirondacks. We went there for our honeymoon back in 2013 and were grateful for the chance to return. My family joined us a couple of days after we arrived, and we all spent a great few days hiking and enjoying the Olympic-related activities, including touring the ice rink where the "Miracle on Ice" hockey game was played, going for a ride in the gondola up Whiteface Mountain, touring the ski-jump facilities, and, coolest of all, riding in a bobsled. Times like that helped remind me that the intensely difficult treatment I was going through was worth it, allowing me more opportunities to live both longer and more richly.

It was a strange time, a summer when I felt mostly all right often enough to do the things I wanted, but also punctuated by some incredible lows. The only time I ever thought I wanted to die came during this summer, and it wasn't a result of any cancer treatment or side effect. It came from opioid withdrawal.

I switched too quickly from one painkiller to another after my stent removal and laparoscopic chest surgery. On paper, there is no reason I would have experienced withdrawal symptoms, but I did. I don't know how anyone can expect a person who is actually addicted to any opioid, especially higher doses than the small amount of hydromorphone I was on, to ever kick the habit. Just switching medications and going down in dosage too quickly was enough to make me feel like I was dying and wish I could get it over with already. I was freezing hot, sweaty and cold, shivering and exhausted. My head felt enormous and inflated but also filled with lead. I wanted to kick and punch and shout and scream, and to curl up in the fetal position and never move a muscle again. It was the most intensely terrible experience I have ever been through or can imagine. And I say that as someone who has been through a lot of terribly difficult cancer treatments.

This experience scared me into getting off my post-operative pain-killers as quickly as possible. I also hate the fuzzy-headedness that comes with strong painkillers, and that too has motivated me to wean off of them shortly after every surgery. Even simple things like a game of Ticket to Ride become all but impossible for me when I'm on drugs like hydromorphone, since such games involve decision-making and arithmetic past the number 20, which for whatever reason becomes my barrier on such medications. But far more than the annoyances of a clouded mind, the fear of addiction and the knowledge of how impossible it could become to get off opioids drove me to wean off them as quickly as I could stand.

I've gotten good at listening to my body, and I've pushed it a little too far and started to experience withdrawal symptoms a couple times, but when that happens the solution is fairly simple: I just take a pill and wean a little slower. Always in the back of my mind lingers the knowl-edge of how easy it would be to grow dependent, how impossible it could become to quit. It has given me an intense empathy for those involved in the ongoing opioid crisis or caught up in any other substance addiction, and it confounds me that we primarily criminalize hard drug use rather than treat it as a health issue.

By now you may have the idea that my cancer treatments have been tough. This is an understatement. They've been downright hellish, in fact, and because I don't like to think about everything I've endured, I'm sure I've downplayed exactly how difficult it has been. It's been really, really difficult.

Like most people of any faith going through something tough, I prayed during it all. I prayed a lot. But not how or when you might think.

Prayer is weird.

I don't know exactly what I think about prayer. I know I covet prayers, and I know I cannot help saying prayers at times. But I don't feel like I understand what they actually accomplish. I've had a complicated relation-ship with prayer my whole life, and particularly during the last few years. I pray plenty, but not often at the times when people traditionally pray in Western Christianity. I've never much liked the way we pray. It feels so impersonal, so formulaic.

"Dear God, thank you for the food, thank you for the weather, please help with this that and the other thing. In Jesus' Name, Amen."

That doesn't feel like conversation. It doesn't feel like it makes much of a difference. Maybe it doesn't. I'm out of the habit of praying before I eat. I should be thankful for my food, and I am, but I don't often pray before I eat. At least half the time, any prayers of mine concerning food come while I'm eating, and those prayers simply beg God to let me get my meal down, have it stay down, or not send me to the bathroom inconveniently, urgently, or for a ridiculous amount of time. And especially all three.

Often, my prayers during cancer treatment have been simple cries for help: "Let me at least get to a trash can before I throw up." "Please let me get through this," whether "this" is a day of feeling chemo-y, an outing I'm certain I'm too fatigued to handle, or another lap around the inpatient unit following yet another surgery. In a lot of ways, these kinds of prayers are my way of asking for my daily bread.

"Help me get to a bathroom without shitting myself" is one of my most common prayers. "Just let me get to a bathroom, God. Just let me get to a bathroom." I've repeated that phrase over and over in a hundred situations and places, from walking in New York City to standing in line at theme parks to being in the comfort of my own place as I leap out of bed and dash to the bathroom. It's the closest thing to a motto that I have. My prayer life frequently feels like a constant barrage of begging just to get through life. It feels a little better than griping to God constantly, complaining all the time, but it hardly seems ideal either.

It's not my only prayer, though, even if it is my most common one. Sometimes, when I feel either very weak or very strong, I pray for healing for myself. I don't even know what that means most of the time. How do I pray to a God of Healing when there's little hope that I will ever be cured? When I don't even know what "cured" would look like for me? What does it mean to ask God to heal me when I don't expect it or believe it will come? I simply don't know. I don't know what it means to ask God for healing. I just don't.

I believe God *could* heal me, but that isn't the same as believing God *will*. I don't think God intervenes miraculously very often, and I see no reason why I'm so special that God would step in on my behalf. I won't complain or question God if God does intervene miraculously and I find myself cured of cancer. But I'd be genuinely surprised, and I'd have to take issue with God healing me miraculously when there are so many other more "deserving" people out there who are dealing with much worse. I don't know what I think about it all.

The only thing I know with certainty about prayer is that I already have the gift of God's Spirit. I think a good portion of how I've handled my own cancer diagnosis so well is due to prayer. I know there are hundreds of people praying for me, and there's a good chance that the peace I've felt about my cancer, peace that has transcended my own reason and understanding, has been at least in part a result of those prayers and God's Spirit at work. Whether or not I get a miraculous healing or anything else I might ask of God, God gives me what I need through the Spirit; as such, I can handle whatever comes of my cancer, be it healing or death, with the certainty that God is with me and I will be with God in heaven sooner or later.

I might be blessed to experience profound peace about my own cancer, but such bliss does not extend to my attitude toward prayer. Sometimes I question everything about prayer and healing. Sometimes I fall into some of the dangerous ways of thinking that I know are wrong but can't quite seem to escape. Sometimes I wonder, "What if I had more faith? What if I asked God for healing and fully believed it would come? What if I still have cancer because my faith isn't deep enough?" A lot of churches teach this sort of thinking. Perhaps they have a point. Many Christians believe that those who don't receive healing from God didn't believe strongly enough. Sometimes I'm tempted to think this. Sometimes I want an easy out of my cancer treatment. I want to believe God will heal me, to ask God for healing, and to be healed.

But I can't, because that isn't the way I see the world working around me or how I experience God at work. I see people with enormous faith who go unhealed. I see people of no faith who have no need of healing in the first place. I know I have an unshakable faith in God, both in God's existence and in my idea about who and what God is. I have many deep, troubling doubts about the more nitty-gritty theological details, but never about the idea or existence of God as I understand God. Shouldn't that be enough to bring healing, if faith is all it takes? Evidently not.

What about Lazarus? I assume he's dead again by now. What about all the apostles and, now that I think of it, every Christian who has ever died? Did all their faith run out eventually? If they had enough faith, why weren't they all healed of whatever illness or injury could afflict them and eventually kill them? If the idea that faith is all that is required for healing is true, then what's to stop anyone with enough faith from attaining immortality here on earth? What would keep a truly faithful person from continually getting healed of any threats to their life indefinitely? But faith as a means to living on earth forever is never a claim made by anyone in Christianity—even with the most cynical reading of Scriptures like John 11:25-26. Living forever is also very far from the point of the Christian faith.

Christianity isn't about benefiting ourselves. It isn't a key to a better life or a religion of health, wealth, and prosperity. It's about the first becoming last, serving and caring for the least among us, taking up our crosses daily as we strive to follow God's guidance and direction. Christianity compels its followers to selflessness and sacrificial love, not to self-seeking attempts at benefiting ourselves.

Jesus never promises health to his followers if they simply believe deeply enough. I said earlier that poor health isn't the result of a moral or faithful failure. To say that we just need enough faith in order for healing to be ours pollutes the teachings of Jesus and ignores the realities of our world. It adds another layer of guilt on the shoulders of the sick, this time telling them that their illnesses could be gone if they were only a little more faithful. It's an idea I reject utterly, even if I still find myself wondering about it at times, wishing it could be true, since it would be so much easier.

As it is, I pray for healing anyway. But I can't pray that way all the time. I need other people to pray for me. It feels selfish to ask for so much for myself all the time, to ask every day for healing when so many other people are suffering far worse. Sometimes a month or two go by when I don't ask God for healing even once. I don't like that anymore than constantly begging and bugging God to heal me, but at least I'm not being monotonous. It brings up a more serious point related to prayer and suffering. Often, we who need prayers need them to come from others. We need other people to cover for us when we're burned out, when we can't bring ourselves to ask for the same thing without hope one more time, when we want to ignore our sickness for a little while and focus on other things, when praying for healing would only remind us of what we need to escape, however briefly.

We who are sick desperately need our faith communities to pray for us when we cannot pray for ourselves. We also need our church families to partake in God's call to heal the sick, whatever that may look like. I've had people lay hands on me and pray. I've been anointed with oil twice, and with water from the Grotto of Lourdes in France once. I've had incense burned for me before my first major surgery. I've been prayed for and thought of by people from a range of religions or none at all. I've wanted all of that. In fact, I've needed all of that, even if I don't know what good any of it does. But here I am, alive today, so who knows.

I won't discount the possibility that some part of my survival is thanks to God's healing and life-sustaining powers. I also won't pretend that prayer alone would ever be enough to keep me alive or that forgoing modern medical treatment in favor of religious-based healing rituals would be a wise idea. Yet the fact remains that I have needed, wanted, and benefited— if only as a placebo—from such practices. I have no doubt that prayers and faithful requests for healing help, even if I have no idea how they do or how much they do.

All the prayers in the world could never be enough for me, though. Not if that's all I got. Prayers are great, but people need more than prayers. I think we as the Church too often use prayer as an excuse for inaction. We use it to feel like we've done something when all we've done is quiet our consciences. Maybe that's too cynical. Maybe I'm underestimating the power of prayer, but I haven't personally encountered a situation where a serious issue was solved by prayer alone without human action working in tandem, but that's my own context, my own life experiences. I could be wrong.

Let's explore the idea of prayers and actions, and how they should perhaps work together. Most people aren't in a position to do much more than think of and pray for me, and that already is more than I would ask of anyone. So there's nothing wrong with offering solidarity, thoughts, prayers, good vibes, or whatever other intangibles one wants to direct at another, whatever the situation. I don't mean to sound like people shouldn't think of or pray for unfortunate circumstances, but a problem arises when thoughts and prayers are all people offer. More specifically, the trouble comes when people who are in a position to offer more give only thoughts and prayers.

During any of my now-traditional Spring Tumor Resection Surgeries, held every March three years running, I didn't want you (unless you're my surgeon) to do my surgeries. I did want you to remember that I was having surgery and pray for it to go well. That's because you (probably) are not my surgeon. You aren't in a position to do more than think of and pray for me. That's fine. But if my surgeons had said, "We're thinking of you and praying for you," and then decided that was enough and they should not even try surgery, I would have been upset, and justifiably so. They at least should try something. There may not be a huge chance that the surgeries would be successful, and as I'm writing this I still don't know if my current treatment is effective. But at least trying every course of treatment is better than doing nothing at all. We're thinking and praying for the best, and we can't do much more than that. But my surgeons can, and they have tried in earnest to solve the problem posed by my tumors—to use their talents, intellect, training, and station in life to keep cancer from killing me. My oncologists can, and they have offered chemotherapy, radiation therapy, and clinical trials to try to kill my cancer.

We see this idea manifest itself in a range of areas. Those who could and should do something offer thoughts and prayers and little else, and I think it sours people on the idea of religion in general and Christianity specifically, since that's the most dominant religion in America. Thoughts and prayers without sufficient action cast Christianity as a pointless belief system that offers platitudes rather than meaningful efforts, and it hurts to see Christianity used as an excuse not to act justly.

When the latest mass shooting happens, everyone offers thoughts and prayers and little else. Meaningful, common-sense regulations seem impossible to come by. When a natural disaster strikes, many people send their "thoughts and prayers" even as we ignore underlying issues like climate change, bad zoning regulations, and overdevelopment of low-lying areas. "Thoughts and prayers" become meaningless words offered to people who—much as they may need consideration and prayer—need tangible, real-world help like shelter, food, and basic safety.

Even miracles don't come about by thoughts and prayers alone. Not in my experience, at least. And in the Bible, miracles tend to be precipitated by faithful action as well. Namaan, though he wanted a quick and easy cure for his leprosy, was only healed after bathing in the Jordan River seven times. A paralyzed man's friends break through a roof to lower him down to Jesus that he might be miraculously healed. Lepers follow Jesus' instructions to show themselves to the high priest and are healed as they go on their way. A woman jostles through a crowd for a chance to touch Jesus' clothes and be healed. Faithful actions are as much or more a part of the solutions to our problems as thoughts and prayers. Thoughts and prayers are only as good as the actions we think about, pray about, and ultimately do.

Let me say again that thoughts and prayers are fine. They're great, actually. I covet the thoughts, prayers, and whatever else people might send my way. I truly need them. The many ways people have let me know I'm thought of and prayed for have made all the difference over the last few years. So thoughts and prayers are great—but not if that's all we get from people who can and should do more.

After all, Jesus didn't say, "I was naked and you thought about how cold that would be in the winter, and you prayed that I would find clothes. I was hungry and you thought about how glad you were that your own stomach was full, and you prayed I'd find some food from that nearby dumpster. I was in jail and you thought about how difficult it must be in prison, felt bad for me, and prayed I'd have visitors." The truly uncomfortable part of this for me is that truthfully, all of us can do more than just think of and pray for someone or some situation. Specifically, *I* can do more.

I need to think about what I can do and pray for the courage to do it. And then I need to do it.

We all—me as much as anyone else who claims to follow Christ—need to be open to the ways we can and should help others, and the ways we can influence the systems around us to help others as well. It might not be popular or easy to think like that, but it's what following Jesus requires. And it's something I'm sure I fail at every single day, even more than I fail at remembering to simply pray for the needs of others.

Chapter 5

Insidious Problems and Implicit Prejudices

August of 2015 brought another surgery, this time to take out my ileostomy bag, look through my abdomen for more tumors, and install a small drain tube for use in a clinical trial. The ileostomy takedown meant the return of going to the bathroom conventionally, which I still regard with mixed feelings. I love being free of the bag; it was annoying, messy, and painful at times. However, it also allowed me to eat whatever I wanted without worrying about when and where I'd be able to go to the bathroom. There are times, even now more than three years later, when I miss that convenience.

The clinical trial I decided to take part in started next. I use the word "decided," but it wasn't much of a choice in my mind. On day one, I signed up for anything and everything available that might help kill my cancer. Plus, I'm happy to take part in any clinical trial that might help those who come after me.

As I understand it, the theory behind my Phase I clinical trial was to use specific protein markers on my tumors' cells to send a small, targeted amount of radiation specifically to those cells. To do this, I needed a drain installed—a small, flexible white tube sticking out of my tummy that meant I could only lie on my right side to sleep.

Starting a couple of days after surgery, I had to pump increasing amounts of saline fluid into the drain tube. The trial itself would involve pumping two liters of radioactive fluid into my abdomen, so I had to spend a week or so stretching my abdomen to make sure the radioactive fluid used in the trial would be able to flow through and hopefully come into contact with any cancer cells that might be hiding in my body. At first, the contents only filled a small syringe, the same kind used to flush IVs. I would flush it into the drain, wait an hour, and see if any drained out. The amount increased to fill a bigger and bigger syringe full of fluid and then an IV bag, and soon I could feel the fluid uncomfortably pushing on me from the inside. By the time I reached two liters, I could barely stand the hour-long wait, even though I spent it watching Parks and Recreation or playing Minecraft, trying to distract myself from the profound discomfort.

The day of the actual trial dose was even harder. The live, radioactive fluid was injected into my abdominal drain, and then I had to lie on my back, left side, stomach, and right side for fifteen minutes each. Lying face-down was the hardest, since my belly was painfully full of fluid. The hope was that changing positions every fifteen minutes for an hour would help the fluid slosh around and reach every area possible. It's difficult to determine the effectiveness of this trial. If it successfully targeted and killed cancer cells, we don't know about them because they died, but it's likely the process accomplished something. I haven't followed up on the status of this trial, though I know I was one of the last people to be part of Phase I, and it's now in Phase II.

I had a couple weeks off before I started conventional radiation therapy, so Christina and I got a golden retriever puppy we named Nutmeg. He's adorable and perfect and a bit clingy due to his owners periodically abandoning him for a day or a month at a time, as he sees it. We debated whether to wait until our lives were more stable and I didn't have to go to New York City for unspecified amounts of time with no warning or pattern. If we had waited, though, we'd still be waiting. We are grateful that we decided to go ahead and get him. He brings a lot of joy to both of us.

Next came one of the weirdest and increasingly difficult phases of treatment for me: abdominal radiation. It started off easy. Christina and I liked my radiation oncologist, which made this treatment a far less daunting prospect. Competent and encouraging, she balanced honesty with positivity in a way that encouraged us but didn't give us false hope or rosy expectations. After meeting with the radiation oncologist, the next steps involved making a mold for me to lie in during treatment and letting the specialists give me some tattoos.

The mold was comfortable. Making it involved the same technology used to custom-fit seats in Formula One cars, which I think is cool. The mold started as a giant plastic bag that they filled with two different liquids. The liquids quickly foamed and bubbled as they reacted. They had me lie on the plastic bag; it got warm as the foam frothed up, and then it started to cool as the foam hardened. It took half an hour at most, and by the end of it I had a durable tub that perfectly fit my body and would help me lie in exactly the same position during each radiation treatment in the coming month.

Next, I laid in the brand new foam mold during a CT scan. This way, the radiology team had a more precise picture of the location of my internal structures when I was lying in the mold, they could tailor how much radiation to send where, targeting areas of concern and avoiding blasting vital organs.

Finally, I got tattoos. The tattoos are tiny dots used to ensure that my position is exactly the same for each dose of radiation. I know where they are, so I can still find most of them, but they're so small I don't think anyone would notice them. They're less prominent than a mole or a freckle, for sure. To get them, right after the CT scan I stayed in my mold, and the technicians turned on an array of lasers that crisscrossed my abdomen. After a few moments spent positioning everything precisely, they marked with a Sharpie where the lasers intersected on my stomach and sides as well as on the mold I was lying in. Then they took a shockingly large syringe filed with ink and gave me eight tattoos, four down the middle of my stomach and two on each side.

After another week or so, the radiology team had put together their plan for my treatment, and it was time to start. I got radiation for about twenty minutes a day, five days a week, for four weeks. It was by far the easiest treatment I could imagine. I felt great. I didn't need my port accessed, my blood counts didn't drop, and the treatment only took a small amount of time each morning, leaving the rest of the day free to enjoy being in New York City. At least at first.

All I had to do was take off my shirt, lie in my comfortable, custom-fit mold, and listen to music while a big machine slowly revolved around me. Sometimes it seemed that I could feel a little heat or intensity coming from the machine, but that may have just been in my mind. Some days it took longer to get me positioned correctly than it did to receive the actual administration of radiation. The radiation machine used a surprisingly simple yet elegant design. It emitted a steady beam of radiation, which was screened through a series of lead rods that moved almost continuously as the machine circled around me. In this way, the beam of radiation that reached me precisely targeted exactly what my radiation oncologist wanted to hit and only minimally affected what she wanted to avoid. The twenty or so minutes spent lying there waiting gave me time to think, and I worked out a lot of the major plot details in the book I was working on during radiation.

Then, about halfway through the treatment cycle, I started to feel worse. And worse. By the last couple days of radiation treatment, I could barely lie flat for twenty minutes before rushing to a bathroom to vomit. I ate less and less, feeling steadily more ill. Once treatment was over, I simply wanted to sleep and mindlessly watch TV and nothing else. I wanted to get through the day as quickly as possible until, hopefully, at some future time, I would feel better.

Radiation was the last step in my original treatment plan. By that point it had been a full year since I was diagnosed, which is how long they said all the treatments they wanted to try would take. We didn't know what would come next, and I wasn't thinking about it at the time. I was focused more on attempting to eat minuscule portions of food and keep it down, trying to kill time and get through another day, and all the while hoping that the next day would be better. I remember thinking that it was strange to have finished all my planned treatment and yet to feel consistently worse than I did since my first rounds of rough chemo—at least, other than the few hours of opioid withdrawal.

Recovery from radiation progressed agonizingly slowly. I could discern no difference from one day to the next. I remember looking back five days or a week later and seeing some progress, but there was no noticeable improvement over the course of just a day or two. It was frustratingly slow and made me think at the time that radiation might be the worst part of my treatment. Sure, chemo has stronger effects and makes them known almost immediately. Yes, major abdominal surgery is far tougher, but not for nearly as long. Radiation, by comparison, is an insidious and sneaky little bugger.

All I did was lie there on a table while a big, fancy machine slowly circled me. It's not like I was cut open from sternum to pelvis or pumped full of poison. I just had to hold still. Nothing even touched me. The first week or two, I couldn't have even told you if the machine was truly emitting radiation or if it was just a placebo. But a month came and went after I finished radiation, and I was still barely able to eat. Sometimes I thought I felt well enough, and I'd eat close to a reasonable portion before feeling horrible, throwing up, and swearing off food for a while. I can tell you in no uncertain terms that yes, my insides were most definitely getting zapped, even if I saw no effects for the first couple of weeks.

Compared to chemo, where a good night's sleep would often considerably lessen the side effects, the healing process for radiation therapy inched along. I remember feeling about the same three weeks after the end of radiation as I did four or five days after surgery. By that time, I ate the same amount of food and felt about as sore in my stomach. At least with radiation there was no NG tube, staples, IVs, or epidurals to deal with, and I tried to be grateful for that. But when my stomach felt perpetually sour and I nearly threw up just thinking about food, life wasn't easy.

I began to wonder what things in my life are like radiation therapy. It's an imperfect analogy. Like any comparison, I can only take it so far. Chemotherapy, surgery, and radiation have all saved my life, and I am immensely grateful for the level of medical care I have received the last few years. With this analogy, I am focusing on treatments and their immediate side effects, not their long-term, life-saving effects.

What, in life, is like radiation therapy? Certainly there are obvious "chemos" and "surgeries" in our lives—those blatantly unhealthy or destructive habits or practices we all have that can so clearly damage our lives, our relationships, our souls. Holding on to hatred, failing to forgive, becoming enslaved to money or food or power are not so difficult to see, even in our own lives, which are of course much harder to examine than the lives of others. These kinds of habits and their consequences are hard to miss, like a surgery that leaves scars or an infusion of chemo that makes you feel terrible within minutes. But what about the radiation therapies, the insidious, sneaky little buggers that we don't realize are happening until damage is already done?

As my wife could tell you, my "radiation" is comfort mingled with laziness. If it's easier not to go out of my way or do something thoughtful, ten times out of nine that's the course I'll take. That's not a typo, by the way. If it's easier to sit and read or watch a movie for three hours than it is to talk to someone and invest in a relationship, that's what I will do. There's nothing wrong with reading a good book or spending a lazy evening watching TV. Those activities wouldn't compare, in most people's minds, to holding a grudge or stopping at nothing to gain more power and influence, no matter how many people get trampled on your way up. But that is why such things are sneaky.

Like lying on a radiation table while a machine moves around you and nothing noticeable happens to your body, a lazy afternoon seems harmless. And, if it doesn't happen too often, it *is* harmless and even good. If I had only gotten one or two days of radiation therapy, I would hardly have the same struggles I faced after twenty days of treatments. When we make habits of wasting time or of putting merely acceptable activities ahead of truly meaningful investments of our time, the long-term effects can become just as painful for us as the consequences of more obvious wrongdoings. It's something I know I need to work on, though feeling genuinely unable to do much more than sit around all day has been the perfect excuse for me to make every day a lazy one, a day when I spend far too much time doing just okay things and nowhere near enough time doing anything meaningful. I know it's a balance, and I know it's not fair to always expect yourself to be productive, but I don't tend to go overboard on that end. I'm more inclined to waste time doing nothing terrible but nothing good either. I plan to work on it, though. Tomorrow. When I'm feeling better. Or so I keep telling myself.

During my radiation treatment, my hair began to regrow. That's a weird thing about cancer treatment. It isn't like most people think, where being bald is synonymous with having cancer and regrowing it is a sure sign of being cured. During the last few years, I've lost, regrown, lost, and regrown my hair more times than I can recall. When I first wrote this in 2017, I had it back, at least for the time being. But now in 2018, a year after I wrote the first draft of this book and as I'm editing it a final time, my hair is gone again.

Before my ordeal with cancer started, I—like most people—assumed that people undergoing cancer treatment did not have hair and that their hair coming back meant they were cured. Now, though, I'm aware that there is no such thing as being "cured" with regard to cancer and that we cannot judge someone's treatment progress by their (lack of) hair. Even so, it can be hard to remember.

For the first few rounds of chemo—more than three years ago now—I kept my hair. I shaved it off preemptively, thinking that I'd lose it right away when treatment began. Then we arrived in NYC and found out it wouldn't go anywhere until later rounds of more intense chemo. So there I was with my hair buzzed short for no real reason. It wasn't even starting to fall out. When it finally went, it was surprisingly quick to come back, often making valiant efforts between rounds of chemo. In July of 2015, only six months into my treatments, I had a full head of hair and a weirdly soft black beard. I looked pretty swarthy and dashing, I must say. People often assumed I was done with treatment, though in truth I had another surgery, chemo, and two kinds of radiation planned, with a couple years more to come that weren't yet planned. As annoying as it might have been to have people I assume I was done and even congratulate me, I couldn't blame them. It's terribly confusing.

I too have made assumptions on the progress of others' treatment based on their hair. I can clearly remember in the late spring of 2015 being glad to see that one of the young patients we had gotten to know had her hair again. I stupidly assumed she was simply back for a follow-up appointment. Sadly, my assumption based on her appearance was horribly wrong. She was merely between treatments, which allowed her hair to regrow. Her cancer had in fact returned, and to a terrible extent. Her situation was the single most heart-wrenching part of my cancer treatment. More than my own cancer ever could, her cancer made me doubt my beliefs and question if I was too flippant or uncaring in my views on cancer and its place in the world. When she passed in 2016 at the age of six, I was shaken far more than I could ever be by my own diagnosis. I was grateful that we at least were passing through Southern California at the time and I was able to leave a note at her memorial, but I don't know what good that does for anyone who has lost a child.

My point is that even I, despite having experienced hair loss and regrowth during ongoing treatment, have made false assumptions about other people's cancer treatment based on their hair. I, as much as anyone, should know that having hair (or not) is not a reliable indicator of treatment progress. My experiences of misjudging other people's cancer based on their hair highlighted for me just how shallow we often are. Western culture emphasizes physical appearance so much that we quickly evaluate and make assumptions based on looks alone. Cancer provides a great example of this. We see someone who is bald and thin and assume they have cancer; when we see that their hair has come back, we presume that they are better. Without knowing a person well and taking the time to understand their situation, we can easily draw the wrong conclusions, even if we have lived through the same situation, even if we have found ourselves on their end of those false assumptions. And these assumptions are everywhere.

We need to realize that we all can unwittingly play host to insidious problems like implicit prejudice. Nearly everyone who claims otherwise is likely either ignorant or dishonest (primarily with themselves). I don't think I know anyone who can truly say they never make a judgment about others based on their appearance. It might be a judgment on someone's health based on how much hair they have, or how rich or poor they might be based on the clothes they wear or the car they drive. It's easy and most of the time I think it's a sort of default setting we have, to make a quick assessment of someone based on their appearance. And that can be very problematic.

I don't mean to suggest that we can blind ourselves to the way others look or even that we should; judging whether or not we need to help someone based on their appearance isn't necessarily a bad assessment to make. But too often our judgments aren't based in fact, and too often we attach value to the judgments we make, viewing people as greater or lesser depending on our impression of their appearance.

So while it's easy to see someone regrowing their hair and assume they're on the road to recovery from cancer, while it's quicker to make snap judgments based solely on how others appear, such assessments rarely reflect the truth and are based in our own biases rather than facts. Most people tend to be biased about hair, thinking those with a "healthy head of hair" are, well, healthy, and people with less hair are perhaps ill. More troubling by far are biases people hold about gender or race that cloud their perceptions and sway their appearance-based judgments.

Recognizing our own implicit biases, whether we make negative or positive assumptions based on someone's appearance, seems like a critical first step toward fixing some of the problems of bias and prejudice that plague this world. It's a process I've only really only started since my diagnosis, in large part because I've seen too many false assumptions made about me or other cancer patients based solely on their appearance. I share this mainly in the hope that others needn't endure a wake-up call like I did to start confronting their own unwitting biases. After all it is the unacknowledged, unseen prejudices that can at least be addressed with education and greater self-awareness.

One experience during my cancer treatment hammered home the idea that we all constantly make judgments based on appearances. One day in the midst of another round of chemo, a powerful realization came over me. For anyone looking at me, it would not be apparent that anything was amiss with my health. Nobody would have known I had several pounds of tumors in my body or just how fragile my life was. That struck me pretty hard.

I used to be an embarrassingly pretentious, judgmental jerk. I still am sometimes, and I'll always have room for improvement. Before cancer, far more often than I'd like to admit, I used to assume that I knew enough about someone from a quick first impression to scoff at them, judge them, or think disparagingly about them or their actions. I'd judge people I thought were trying too hard to fit in, or not trying hard enough, or who couldn't control their dogs, or any number of other silly things. Driving poorly around me was—and remains—a good way to get me to judge you, both as a driver and, more unfairly, as a human. Less obviously problematic, I might see someone who looks healthy and assume that they are, or I might assume someone is as rich or poor as they appear.

As such, I'll always remember one day early in my treatment. I walked hand-in-hand with Christina back to the Ronald from the hospital and caught the seemingly envious stare of a guy about my age passing the other way. I suddenly realized that anyone could easily look at us and judge us wrongly, even to the point that they would covet my life. That would be ridiculous. Nobody should be jealous of *my* life, I thought. I have cancer, for crying out loud, and if anyone knew that, surely they'd pity me, not envy me. More clearly than ever before, I saw that assuming things about people based on a first impression is dangerous and unhealthy.

Then I realized I had two things to learn.

First, when I stop to think about it, there are actually plenty of potential reasons for others to be jealous of my life. While my life may not be perfect, and while I would willingly trade a great deal to be healthy and cancer-free for many, many years, I also have plenty for which I am grateful. I have a lot going for me, and, cancer aside, I live a charmed and privileged life. Maybe it isn't so absurd, after all, to think that someone might be jealous of my life.

Second, considering what others might conclude when seeing my wife and me happily strolling along together highlighted the main problem with assuming I know anything about anyone just by looking at them. To look at us then, you might never have suspected that I was in the midst of brutal cancer treatments. It was cold and I wore a winter hat, hiding my baldness. If you knew what the Memorial Sloan Kettering Pediatric Day Hospital logo on the back of my blue backpack meant, or noticed the IV tube going from the bag into my body, you might have had a hint that not all was well with me, but I doubt most people notice things like that. For pretty much all appearances, Christina and I looked like a typical, happy, healthy couple, even in the midst of the hardest chemo. Certainly, to look at me now, even when I'm bald (as long as I have my eyebrows), you'd likely never suspect I was anything but healthy—at least if I keep my shirt on, hiding my surgical scars. I'm shockingly skinny, but for all you know I could just be a long-distance runner. (Please note: I am *not*.)

This lesson has stuck with me. I don't know just from looking at anyone what their story may be, where they are in life, or why they're doing what they're doing. I should have realized that earlier, but it wasn't until I could see that principle applied so clearly to myself that I actually took it to heart. It appears throughout the Bible too: "Let anyone among you who is without sin be the first to throw a stone" (John 8:7); "Do not judge, so that you may not be judged" (Matt 7:1-2). Jesus even singled out our predilection for making assumptions based on looks, imploring us to "not judge by appearances, but judge with right judgment" (John 7:24). These passages are hardly new to me, but I never understood their lesson until recently—at least not enough to take them to heart in a truly meaningful way.

Someone who looks healthy could be just like me and have recently made it through a long period of hellish cancer treatment. They could even have cancer that has yet to be discovered. Perhaps the reason some bad driver I'm angry with is on the phone while drifting out of his lane is that he's currently receiving terrible news over the phone as he drives. He should still pull over and not endanger his life and the lives of those around him, but not everyone can think clearly in crises, so I should cut people some slack.

Assuming anything based on clothing the way I used to (and sometimes still do) is wrong too. Someone could be impoverished and wearing the one nice set of clothing she owns as she heads to an interview for a job she desperately needs. Or, conversely, she might be wealthy and wearing grungy clothing because she's been doing manual labor. That gruff cashier or angry patron could be coping with loss or abuse or any number—other than zero—of terrible problems. Who knows? Not me. The point is, without knowing someone's full story, without understanding the whole situation, it is impossible to say what is really going on. It is impossible to judge the people or the situation, even if it were my job to do so, which it is not.

Cancer has taught me to give people more grace and not to concern myself with all the little things other people do that I might not agree with or that I find annoying. They could have a good reason for their actions. They might not. It doesn't matter as much as I used to think. Unless I get to know someone and understand their circumstances, I cannot even begin to judge them fairly. And once I do know someone, once I understand everything they're going through, I really won't want to judge them at all.

Chapter 6

Planning the Unplannable

By Thanksgiving—five weeks after the end of my radiation treatment—I was able to eat a little. Not much, but at least enough to have a couple bites of turkey and some mashed potatoes. We spent that thanksgiving down in Tallahassee, Florida, at Christina's parents' place. They are truly lovely, generous people who have supported us immensely during my cancer treatment in a dozen ways. They steadfastly prayed for us and gave financially to us, helped move our things to Corning when I was first diagnosed, visited us or invited us over numerous times, facilitated an amazing trip to the incredible Universal Studios and Islands of Adventure theme parks in Orlando, bought me a remote-control helicopter small enough to fly inside my room at the Ronald, and remain all-around sources of encouragement for Christina and me. We both owe them greatly, and they're a significant part of making my whole experience with cancer go as well as it has.

I had my first abdominal fluid buildup while I was recovering from radiation treatment. It isn't particularly common as a side effect, so it was concerning enough to warrant draining the fluid and sending it off for a biopsy, but it returned negative for any cancer cells, a huge relief. I also had another PET/CT scan during this time. I, of course, had several others during treatment to see if my chemo was having any kind of effect on my tumors, to plan for surgeries, to see the results of surgeries, and so on. But this was the first scan that had the potential of being clear of any signs of cancer.

It wasn't.

It wasn't particularly definitive either way, which is better than an obviously terrible scan result, but it wasn't what we hoped for either. Since it was still reasonably close to the end of my radiation therapy, there was a decent chance that the results were skewed from that treatment too. So we scheduled another scan in eight weeks. With scan results that weren't totally clear and the end of my originally planned treatment behind us, we faced some decisions.

My oncologists wanted me to go on maintenance chemotherapy. It would be a much lower dose than the intense drugs I had taken most recently, but, given my intense reaction to the supposedly tolerable, low-dose drugs at the beginning of my treatment, I was wary. I wanted a break. I *needed* a break. I needed to recover more and get stronger. I wanted to be done with cancer, too, but I knew that was wishful thinking. More realistically, I wanted a chance to rebuild some strength before diving back in to more treatment. And I wanted to live a little, free from constant medical care.

Maintenance chemo would require three weeks of chemo with one off week. There was no way to guarantee that I still had cancer and needed maintenance chemo or that this chemotherapy regimen would work if I did. Having been through a year of intense treatment already, I decided it was time for a break. I might start on maintenance chemotherapy later, I might need more surgeries or radiation in the future, but for now, I just wanted to be free from cancer treatments.

We went back to Florida to be with Christina's parents for a month. It was great to spend more time with them and be outside and active. January is a great time to go to Florida. The afternoons aren't as hot and humid as in the summertime, and the evenings are pleasant. I love winter activities like hockey, snowboarding, and skating on the pond up in Corning, but it is undoubtedly easier to stay regularly active when it's 75 degrees Fahrenheit outside instead of 15. Christina's parents live next to the Miccosukee Greenway, a well-maintained trail that feels wonderfully wild and far away from everything despite its proximity to the suburbs. It features a surprising amount of topography too, with gentle hills and a crossing over a seasonal creek bed. The live oaks resplendent with Spanish moss remain my favorite feature of the area, and I was able to go for a walk almost every day. I ate more and more, felt better and better, and even went jogging. It was easy to forget about cancer for a little while.

But all things end, and too soon we found ourselves back in New York City for my follow-up scan. The results came back much the same as before, if not a little worse. It was still more vague and ambiguous than obviously bad, but it certainly wasn't great either. My doctors wanted to follow up in six weeks instead of in three months, as we had hoped.

We already had tentative plans for a road trip out west, and now that we knew how much time we had until my next scan, we narrowed our ideas, deciding on the national parks and places we could realistically enjoy in six weeks. I grew up traveling. Most summers during my childhood, my family went on extended road trips, camping all the way. I figured that was normal. By the time I started eighth grade, I had been to all forty-eight contiguous US states and nine Canadian provinces. The only corner of the country I hadn't explored was the extreme Southwest. I'd been to Santa Fe, the Grand Canyon, and Yosemite before but never to southern New Mexico, Arizona, and California. And I had only passed through the Texas panhandle, which hardly counts as visiting Texas. These factors plus the time of year—it was February and northern areas were still closed for camping due to snow—made the Southwest seem like the logical area to explore.

The first day, we drove about nine hours and nearly made it to South Bend, Indiana. It seemed a weird to me to spend a whole day in the car and end up at home. South Bend, where I lived the first eighteen years of my life, will always be home for me at some level, even as steady changes leave it less recognizable every time I'm back. The cornfields near my old house are all warehouses now. But such is the way of the world, I suppose. It snowed heavily that first night, but not enough to keep me from driving a couple of miles from our hotel to the closest Culver's. (If you've never been to the Midwest, go there just for the Culver's. Order cheese curds and a concrete mixer, even if you're lactose intolerant. It'll be worth it.)

Next, we drove to Lincoln, Nebraska. My older sister, Korynne, was finishing her master's program in cello performance and had an important recital that several relatives came to enjoy. Korynne's recital was brilliant, and after a pleasant few days in Lincoln with her, my parents and grandparents, and some aunts, uncles, and cousins, we headed off westward in a forty-mile-per-hour crosswind. Thankfully our road led us south after a couple of hours, so it became a stiff tailwind that gave us the best gas mileage we've ever gotten from our car, but we were still glad when it finally died down somewhere in Kansas or Oklahoma.

Carlsbad Caverns National Park was our first stop. It was a little too early for the massive swarms of bats that roost in the cave seasonally, but that didn't diminish how impressive it was. I thought Mammoth Cave in Kentucky was big before, but Carlsbad is on another level. Outside the cave, the sunset over the Guadalupe Mountains was spectacular.

White Sands National Monument came next. We stopped there briefly on our way to Arizona. Our golden retriever, Nutmeg, proving he was a northern dog at heart, thought the cool white sand was snow and tried to eat it, but in his defense there were people sledding on the gleaming dunes, and without the heat it could have been a winter's scene. That night we met the first in a line of wonderful campground hosts who made our trip better; she squeezed us into an empty space that wasn't an official campsite at Rockhound State Park, still in New Mexico. Visitors are allowed to keep any rocks they find, so Christina and I went for a short hike and gathered some of the more interesting and colorful stones we saw.

Tucson, Arizona, came next, and with it two surprises. First, Saguaro National Park is exceptionally vibrant, at least in late February. It is undeniably a scorching desert, yet it offers a dazzling variety of plants and shades of green. I looked in vain for a pack of hunting Harris's hawks, but it was hard to be disappointed at not seeing any when there was so much else to absorb. I did get to see one solitary Harris's hawk later that day perched on a fencepost, so the day wasn't a total loss in the birdwatching department. The second surprise in Tucson was Culver's. I'm guessing enough snowbirds from Wisconsin—where the wonderful fast-food franchise originated—winter in Arizona that they've brought their butterburgers with them. Since it soared into the 90s that February day, my wife had no choice but to stop for some frozen custard.

That night we made it to the Phoenix, Arizona area, where my oldest sister, Elyssa, lived at the time. We spent a couple of nights at her place and explored some of the highlights of the area before heading north toward Sedona. We camped, hiked, saw pre-Columbian cliff dwellings, spent an evening in Flagstaff, and hiked some more. Sedona and the surrounding region ranks high on my list of favorite places.

After Arizona, we headed to California. First, we spent a few freezing nights in the unique and splendid Joshua Tree National Park. It was an incredible campground, nestled among giant granite boulders, and we enjoyed hikes, scenic drives, and views of the scenic Coachella Valley from a lofty lookout point. Our next planned stop was Death Valley, but we decided to add a detour through Las Vegas on the way since neither of us had ever been there.

Vegas was not our scene, and the thought of how much money gets gambled away made us sick as we considered how much pediatric cancer research it could fund. I'm glad we stopped there so I know I never want to go there again.

Death Valley National Park was the hottest place we endured on the whole trip. It was only early March, and already temperatures soared above 90. We arrived at the tail end of the wildflower bloom, but there was still a lovely array of different flowers that we could tell were about to disappear, leaving everything desolate, bare rock and sand again.

Finally, we left the desert behind. After a couple weeks of being hot and dry, it was wonderful to get to the Sierra Nevada Mountains, still resplendent in snow, and reach more temperate, wetter climates. Sequoia National Park was next on our list. It snowed at higher elevations the evening we arrived, which meant we set up camp in the rain, but it made the next day all the more incredible. Several feet of snow blanketed the ground higher up where the sequoias grow, and we enjoyed an informative ranger-led snowshoe trek through the groves of massive trees. Sequoia is probably my favorite national park. A few short days were not nearly long enough in this park. A year would not be enough.

San Francisco came next, and Christina's sister Rachel flew out to meet us since it was spring break at the school where she teaches. We packed too much into too little time, but I'm not sure I would change anything if we did it again. After a quick tour of San Francisco, we headed down the coast, stopping at the Monterrey Bay Aquarium where I have wanted to go since I was a kid collecting marine animal toys in their aquarium series. I don't have a formal bucket list, but if I did this would be on it. The aquarium did not disappoint, and from the observation deck we saw a wild baby sea otter with its mom. Experiences like this reassured me that I had made the right choice, and still, looking back on it, I think that taking a break from treatment and going on a crazy road trip of a lifetime was the best decision. If I have to die of cancer, I'm damn sure going to live first.

Continuing down the coast, we were struck continually with the natural beauty of the Big Sur region, camping for a night among soaring redwoods. Even more impressive was the wildlife. I caught a fleeting glimpse of a peregrine falcon stooping toward some out-of-sight prey. We saw sea otters, dolphins, and migrating gray whales, mostly mothers with calves. A pod of humpback whales also passed by as we ate lunch at the aptly named Whale Watcher's Café. But the most interesting fauna we encountered were the elephant seals. I wasn't expecting them, which made them all the more impressive. They apparently breed a little earlier in the year, so it wasn't quite peak season for them, but there were still several hundred of the great hulking beasts lazing around on the beach.

Santa Barbara made for a lovely evening; we got ice cream on the pier, which seemed like the thing to do there. We were short on time, but we still managed to enjoy a few of the local touristy sights in Los Angeles as well, like the Walk of Fame and a cool beach with a small cave that floods when the tide comes in. I won't pretend we weren't typical tourists, gawking at everything as we complained about the traffic.

After Rachel flew back home to Florida, we got a phone call from Sloan Kettering. I don't remember why, but my scans were delayed so we suddenly had an extra week and no longer needed to start the long drive back home right away. So I did what anyone who played Roller Coaster Tycoon in middle school does with extra time in the LA area: I went to Magic Mountain. Then it was time to start heading home, though we had enough spare time for a few quick stops along the way. Starting in LA, we set off on I-10, ready to drive its entire length from coast to coast.

The great part about I-10 once you get into Texas is that the speed limit is 80 miles per hour. The bad part about I-10 once you get into Texas is that it still takes forever to cross the enormous state. We stopped for a couple of nights in San Antonio, seeing the Alamo and the enchanting river walk and spending a day at Six Flags Fiesta Texas. I love roller coasters, and it was fun to be able to visit some theme parks I had never expected to see. The home stretch of our road trip took us from San Antonio to Tallahassee in a single day, with a quick stop in New Orleans for beignets from Café Du Monde, since that's a requirement for tourists in New Orleans.

After a too-short Easter weekend with Christina's family, we drove back to Corning in another long, tiring day. All told, we went through twenty-three states and, according to the trip odometer in our trusty Subaru, drove 9,653.2 miles. I say "we," but I mean "I," since Christina didn't drive once. Not that she was unwilling, but I love driving and she loves being a passenger and is an excellent navigator and co-pilot (no matter what I might say in the heat of the moment when I don't know where I'm going), so the arrangement works out. Give me an open road and the entire Lord of the Rings trilogy on audiobook and I'm good to go. All told, it was an incredible trip, one that wouldn't have happened without my cancer as an incentive to take it.

Then I had my scans. The results weren't great. I needed surgery for some spots on my chest, which they scheduled for the following week. I had always wanted to go skiing at Jay Peak in Vermont and Whiteface Mountain near Lake Placid, so Christina and I headed up there in the meantime. It was early April, so neither place was fully open, but it snowed powder the whole time at Jay, and the long, winding run from the top of the gondola to the bottom of the mountain at Whiteface was exhilarating. If I was going to have surgery in a few days, I decided I wanted to go into the operating room with happy memories and no regrets of things left undone.

I learned a few lessons during this time, perhaps the most wonderful months of my life. First, we have to enjoy life and make plans to do what we really want to do, to complete those activities that we'll forever regret if we leave them untried. Second, we can't plan or control anything. Those two lessons seem contradictory at first, but I have found that they actually work in harmony together.

I'm glad we planned (and improvised!) an awesome road trip to a bunch of places I had long wanted to visit. It might not have been the most responsible choice to take a break from treatment and go on a trip for more than a month. But I don't always want to be responsible. I want to enjoy life. I'm not suggesting that people should fritter away their time and money on whatever seems enjoyable at any given moment, but we need to make sure we actually do the things we want with our lives. If we don't take that vacation, if we don't see that sight, try that activity, live that life, take time to enjoy the good in this world, then what are we really doing? Why am I fighting to stay alive if not, at least in part, to live richly and fully? I haven't always thought this way during my treatment. It took me a while to figure this out, and I still probably get it wrong today more often than I'd like to admit.

Back in December 2014, I was miserable far more often than not. The "easy, low-dose" chemo did *not* agree with me in the slightest—at least, not nearly like the potent stuff did, for whatever reason. With the various unpleasant side effects and symptoms I endured, the low odds of my survival seemed all too believable. I mentioned before how I regarded myself too much as a cancer patient and needed the example of others to make me realize that I could still have fun while going through treatment. But even after I learned to enjoy the present as a cancer patient and try to have fun in the middle of it, I still let cancer consume my plans for the future.

Early in my treatment, I decided to not let myself get too excited about anything in the future, especially anything more than a month or so away. I implicitly assumed I wouldn't be around too far into the future, and honestly, I wasn't sure I wanted to be. Just getting through one day at a time was more than enough to handle.

So when I first heard that a new Jurassic Park movie would release that upcoming summer, I wanted to be excited, but I figured I wouldn't live to see the film. When I watched the trailer and heard the iconic soundtrack, I tried to temper my excitement somehow, telling myself that it probably wouldn't be worth seeing, or something along those lines. That way I wouldn't be too disappointed if I died before the film came out. More logically, I didn't want people to have one more trigger reminding them that I was gone, one more potentially fun activity tainted by the idea that I was missing out on it, or that it would have been more fun if I were there sharing in it. Let's be honest here: I'm pretty much the life of any party!

Then winter turned to spring, and my first surgery went well, and then my second, and then I met Chris Pratt when he visited the Ronald McDonald House that April and got an awesome autographed velociraptor toy. (I promise I'm not 8 years old . . . well, maybe I am a little bit.) I finally decided it was all right to look forward to seeing *Jurassic World*. I would fully allow myself to look forward to the movie, to plan on going, and to tell everyone multiple times how much I wanted to see it the day it opened in theaters.

When opening day finally arrived, we ended up going with one of the larger gatherings of Wisconsin cousins in recent memory, and though the movie could certainly have been better, it was still a lot of fun. But the only reason we were able to get as many of us together as we did is because we planned ahead. It might seem like a small thing, an evening at the movies with cousins, but I don't see it as such. I think it's precisely these types of moments that make life rich and fulfilling. And through that evening at the movies—and a hundred other events like it during my cancer treatment—I've learned that I should never feel that I can't make plans for the future, no matter how unpredictable it may seem.

The future is always uncertain, often even more so than it seems to us. It is our circumstances that force us to realize or, most often, enable us to forget this harsh truth. But rather than refusing to look ahead or dream about what might be for the sake of realism, we should make plans with an asterisk attached, an implied assumption that these plans get a green light IF we stay alive, IF everything goes as we all hope, IF nothing earth-shattering happens between now and then. It shouldn't be a shocking lesson. This idea gets specific mention in James 4:13-15, which tells us that we cannot know the future and shouldn't make plans as if we're totally in control.

Anyone's plans can be easily smashed to bits by the uncertainty of life. Simply using a ladder or crossing a street could alter a person's plans for the future just as easily as cancer could. Interacting with a material world always brings a chance of death. Living life carries an inherent risk of dying. It is only when we get comfortable that we forget just how delicate our lives are and begin to think our plans are set in stone.

I bear a dozen surgical scars reminding me of my mortality, of the futility of planning too far ahead. It's tempting, given my situation, not to bother with plans at all, or at least not with anything beyond the next scan. And in many ways, I can't plan past my next PET/CT scan. There's always a chance I'll need sudden surgery and the next month will get thrown into disarray—and that's okay.

It's the balance that matters. Christina and I have gotten good at figuring out this balance. It's hard to know what perfect planning would look like, especially in our situation, but we're doing all right. We make plans as best we can, not bothering to look too far ahead and remembering when we do that anything beyond the next scan is tentative. But we still plan. We still prepare for the future. We still write in our planner as far ahead as possible, even when it feels pointless to plan for a life far outside our control.

In a lot of ways, that feeling is right. Not much in life is within our control or even falls under our ability to influence. Our culture fosters the illusion of control, and it is easy to forget how little power we have. We plan and schedule our days, we believe our hard work will pay off, and we take for granted that we're living longer than ever. And sure, to an extent we should. It's easy to give up and stop caring about much when you lose some feeling of control. My lack of regard for the future when I first started treatment was deeply unhealthy; believing everything in life will play out as it will regardless of our efforts is too extreme a view in the other direction. So, as I see it, we cannot see the future and we cannot know how our lives will play out, but that fact does not absolve us from being responsible and preparing for whatever may come.

Luke 12 contains a parable that I think relates closely to this idea. The story of the rich fool tells of a man who enjoys a bountiful harvest and in response rebuilds his barns bigger so that he might hoard his grain and goods. Yet just as he is prepared to sit back, relax, and enjoy a life of leisure, God informs him that he will die that very night. "The things you have prepared," God asks of the man, "whose will they be?" (12:20, NRSV). Jesus sums up in Luke 12:21 by saying, "So it is with those who store up treasures for themselves but are not rich toward God" and, by extension, toward the people God would have us serve. It's a parable primarily about selfishness and how we hoard things rather than use them for good, but it's also about the futility of putting off everything for some future day we may not live to see. Both are important lessons I've come to appreciate during my cancer treatment. If we aren't careful, we can become so caught up in planning for the future that we forget to live in the present, like the rich fool who died before enjoying any of his wealth. Similarly, when we don't make a conscious effort to act philanthropically, we easily delay the charitable activities we want to do for some future day when we'll have more time, energy, and money to give. And in my experience at least, we'll never have so much time, energy, and money that we'll feel like we finally have extra to give.

My life, my uncertain grasp on staying alive, makes painfully obvious what is true for us all: none of us knows the future, and we could die at any time. The best any of us can do is not squander the time we have and appreciate every minute for what it's worth. We have to use our lives to serve others now, while we can, and we need to balance planning for an uncertain future with remembering that we are not nearly as powerful as we like to think.

Chapter 7

I Love You, Church, but Sometimes . . .

My laparoscopic chest surgery went smoothly, all things considered. I had to leave my chest tube in for several days afterward, but the fluid draining from me did eventually slow down on its own. Having the tube required me to say in the hospital longer than anticipated, but of all the complications I might have had, this was fairly minor and it resolved itself without further interventions or procedures.

The suspicious nodes that my incredible surgeon removed were indeed cancer. It wasn't surprising, I suppose, but it was still disappointing. There had been a chance that the spots on my scans were merely inflammation of some kind, and however unlikely that might have been, we were still hoping for such results. A small part of me believed I could be done with all my cancer treatment after a full year, even if logically I knew I would likely never be free from the grip of the disease. Since the suspicious spots in my chest had only gotten worse the last couple of months and turned out to be cancer, it was clear I needed more treatment. More radiation therapy came first.

Christina and I met again with my radiation oncologist, this time feeling a bit more cynical, given my difficult experiences with abdominal radiation. But again, the oncologist's honesty about how my past radiation went, coupled with her reassurances that a few weeks of radiation to the chest wouldn't aggravate my entire digestive system like abdominal radiation had, helped calm our nerves. At worst, the radiation therapy they planned for my chest would give me terrible heartburn and some difficulty swallowing, both of which might take some time to resolve but should ultimately prove temporary and manageable.

So I signed on for another round of radiation therapy, this one focusing on my chest. They still had my body mold in storage, which saved time preparing for this new round but also made me wonder how long they keep them and assume people will be back for further treatment. They were also able to use my uppermost tattoos from before, so I only needed three more dots inked into my skin—one on each side and one in the middle of my chest—and then I was set.

Again, all I had to do was lie still as the radiation machine rotated around me. Again, I wondered if I could actually feel a strange sort of "heat" emanating from it or if that was merely a product of my imagination. Unlike my first round of radiation treatment, this phase only lasted two weeks and brought few side effects. I experienced a little heartburn that was easily cured by avoiding acidic foods and taking the occasional antacid. I also had trouble swallowing for about three days, but it wasn't so serious that an extra gulp or two of water couldn't take care of it. This was the easiest phase of my entire treatment. I still think I prefer surgery for its simple, understandable, physical nature over the intangible forces of radiation that defy comprehension and don't produce immediate results, but, if I had to do one phase of treatment over, I'd pick chest radiation. It was the only phase of treatment that I can honestly say was not unpleasant in some way.

By the end of my radiation treatment, it had been more than a year and a half since my diagnosis. Now, more than four years out, that doesn't seem so long, but at the time it seemed like forever. In many ways I don't feel that I can remember what life was like "BC," *before cancer*. Not that everything has disappeared from my memory; I just can't remember my perspective on life from that time or recall what it was like not to live with daily reminders that I am deeply unwell and unlikely to survive this disease. I can't remember what it was like to think of time in increments longer than three months ahead.

A year and a half of living this way started to wear on me—and my wife too. A year and a half of trying every treatment invented, even doing a clinical trial for a treatment still being invented, all in the hope of staving off death a little longer is inherently discouraging, especially after our short break from it all to take a road trip in the Southwest. Now we were forced back into a world we wanted to escape, a world of cancer, unending treatments, and little hope. I cannot begin to imagine how much darker our thoughts would have turned without the support we enjoyed—and still enjoy—from so many people.

Family, friends, and friends of friends have all joined our group on Facebook to follow my treatments. I've had blankets, hats, a year's supply of Stroopwafels, magazines, books, brainteasers, and, yes, money, sent to me from across the country and around the globe. Christina and I have been buoyed by an incredible wave of support, especially early in my treatment when my diagnosis was shocking and our needs were uncertain.

People from a wide range of religious and nonreligious backgrounds have been key components in our support network. We've enjoyed a tremendous amount of support from dozens of people unaffiliated with any Christian church, and that fact is not lost on me. This is, however, a book about cancer and Christianity, and I would be remiss if I didn't dedicate some time to discussing the ways the church has and has not supported us, and indeed the ways it can and cannot support people in situations like mine.

Numerous churches—from the one I grew up in for eighteen years to ones attended by people I have never met—have helped us in dozens of ways. I have been visited and hosted by people from church, upheld in prayer, and anointed with oil. From special offerings collected for us to generous individuals who continue to give to us, we have been helped financially by the incredible generosity of more churches than I can keep track of. In a lot of ways, I could not and would never expect or ask for more support than we've already received.

The church has been far from perfect, and I can't sugarcoat or ignore that fact either. Despite the amazing and ongoing support from individuals, the Church in this country—that is, Christians as a collective whole—have too often fallen short of being the hands and feet of Jesus. From a shocking lack of empathy and support for people in situations like mine to inflammatory statements and hurtful actions regarding the roles of church and government in healthcare, I haven't felt uplifted or encouraged by the Church all the time since becoming a cancer patient.

Sometimes, the Church and people who most loudly claim it as theirs have been the biggest source of discouragement in my life. From mercifully few in-person conversations to far too many online interactions on places like Facebook and Twitter, to the rhetoric from politicians who would bring destructive changes to our healthcare system, I've experienced firsthand what it's like to have Christians suggest I'm morally culpable for my cancer, that the cost of trying to save my life isn't worth others potentially having to pay higher insurance rates, and a slew of other unloving, dehumanizing, and otherwise troublesome statements.

As someone with cancer, I've experienced just a fraction of what it feels like to be marginalized by the church, and it has opened my eyes to the destructive ways that the church I love is oppressing other groups far more than anything I've experienced firsthand. As a straight male, my experiences with Christians who sought to blame me for my cancer have really helped me to empathize more with what it must be like to be female in a denomination that does not allow women to preach, or gay in a church that is not affirming and inclusive.

One idea backed by a lot of Christians that has given me particular grief the last couple of years is the notion that the church, not the government, should take care of the sick. It's one of the more bizarre statements that I've encountered. First, this idea ignores the realities of what it takes to care for the sick in this day and age, and, second, it presents a false dichotomy about the roles of church and government that nobody I know actually believes—at least, not when applied to other issues.

I'll start by agreeing with the first premise in this statement. Yes, the church should and must care for the sick. Jesus makes clear in Matthew 25 that those who provide food to the hungry, drink to the thirsty, hospitality to the stranger, clothing to the naked, care to the sick, and companionship to the imprisoned are considered righteous in God's eyes. The parable of the Good Samaritan too proclaims that it is good and right to care for others, perhaps especially when it is inconvenient and costs us our time, money, or even our own safety. So yes, the church needs to care for the sick. But it doesn't. And it can't—not on its own, at least.

No church I've ever been part of has an extra million dollars per year in its budget for the medical bills of just one member. That's how much my cancer treatment cost the first two years. The third and fourth years have been cheaper, but it's still far more than my current church's entire annual budget. That's why I have insurance; that's why I *need* insurance—insurance that, thanks to current government regulations, can't be cut off for annual and lifetime limits that I would quickly surpass. If caring for the sick were solely the responsibility of the church, people like me with rare and expensive medical conditions would bankrupt churches and quickly end up without access to life-saving treatments. The church can and must tend to the sick, but it also simply cannot pay for everyone's medical care on its own.

Of course, even if medical care were far cheaper or a lot more rich people donated copious amounts of money so that the church could somehow pay medical bills, there would still be no reason that our government should not also play a role in our healthcare system. The idea that it's the church's job and therefore not the government's would still be a false dichotomy. If the church should do *something*—if something is noble and just—why should the government necessarily avoid such things? The only possible answer to this question is that we must have separation of church and state, but that doesn't really apply here. Certainly, no religion should unduly influence our government or insist that its tenets become the law of the land. But that doesn't mean a government should abandon its duties to its citizens—such as providing for the right to healthcare—merely because members of a particular religion also believe in sharing that responsibility and want to help in that area.

I don't think anyone really believes this false dichotomy. Certainly, I don't know anyone who applies this principle consistently. It strikes me as odd that many of the same people who say the government should get out of healthcare because the church should care for the sick also want—for religious reasons—the government to decide who can or can't marry. It is inconsistent to vote for elected officials who promise to bring "Christian" principles to our government while also saying that the government shouldn't do something the church is supposed to do, and I can't fathom the sort of mental gymnastics that make it possible to hold both ideas simultaneously.

I think many Christians are simply embarrassed that our government is doing a better job than the church at systematically providing food for the hungry and giving the sick a way to receive the healthcare they need. I know I am embarrassed. I cannot claim to have made nearly enough effort in such areas as I should, and every time I read Matthew 25:36, a knot ties in my stomach, compelling me to do better, to seek those who need help, and to do my part to share God's love. As it is, I do next to nothing to contribute to these areas myself, and I wish I and the church as a whole were both better examples of Christ's love. Sure, my current health makes reaching out to other ill people difficult, but that's a tepid excuse. I didn't volunteer much before I got cancer. We as the Church can and must do better. If we're embarrassed, as perhaps we should be, we need to change.

How should the church care for the sick while recognizing the government's role in healthcare? First, we must recognize that there are many ways of caring for the sick that the government cannot do. The church can provide community that the government cannot. The church can provide spiritual care that the government cannot. The church can be a source of comfort and strength extending far beyond financial support—though it can and should work to improve its care in that area too. But the church simply cannot provide comprehensive medical coverage for everyone—not with current attendance and financial giving trends. In light of that, we the church should support and encourage our government to work toward healthcare policies that protect the sick and ensure they are cared for, even as we work together to care holistically and spiritually for those facing illness. The church can offer care for the sick. Without church support, I don't know where I'd be financially, mentally, and spiritually. And that's why it hurts so deeply to see the church not living up to its full potential, to see it actually harming others.

If there is a single imperative of Christianity, it is to love. By such a litmus test, I think most of us who claim Christianity fail daily to show ourselves as disciples of Christ, and I want to make it clear that I include myself among the guilty. When I think about the discussions I have been part of recently or the conversations I hear on the national stage, hatred, not love, is the common theme.

Far too often, I've been guilty of harboring hatred in my heart toward individuals rather than toward their words, ideas, or actions. There's a subtle but important difference between a valid criticism of a terrible, unloving idea and an *ad hominem* attack. It is the difference between statements such as "so-and-so *is* a despicable person" and "so-and-so's continued use of hostile, intentionally controversial rhetoric is despicable," or at least "so-and-so's racism is despicable." It is, at the core, the difference between dehumanizing and hating others—the very thing I want to stand against—and remembering that all are made in the image of God and deserve God's love and compassion, even if their ideas and beliefs are reprehensible.

Many people I otherwise agree with claim there's too much hate in the world today not to respond in kind. "Fight fire with fire," I hear people say. Part of me wants to agree with them. I've been tempted to hate the people working to undermine the patient protections in our laws that have saved my life the past few years, like not being discriminated against by insurance companies for having health issues. But that still gives me no right to yell at anyone about politics, to declare that I am completely, absolutely right, and that to disagree with me is to be a misinformed idiot who wants to kill cancer patients.

One thing cancer has taught me is that you never know what someone else might be going through. If someone posts an inflammatory Facebook status about their political views, I should answer their anger and frustration with kindness and love. I should try to ask questions to see how they attempt to defend their indefensible views—and maybe realize they can't—rather than just attack, attack, attack. It may not change their minds, but neither will yelling and name calling. A little compassion might be just what they need.

Besides, fighting fire with fire only works with wildfires if there are thousands of acres to burn and you don't mind leaving vast swathes scorched. It is not a good strategy for combating a house fire, and that's what we're dealing with right now in the church. We can't afford to fight fire with fire, to answer hatred with more hate. If we do that, hatred wins and the whole world will lie charred and desolate. We must extinguish hate with love instead—whatever that means and however that looks at any given moment.

Yes, Jesus flipped tables and shouted, and sometimes there's a time for that. But Jesus also sought out the marginalized and offered them love to counteract the hatred society poured out against them. More to the point, Jesus himself rebuked others with loving, tough questions, not just stern words. I should try to do that as well. We need to ask ourselves how we can smother hatred with a loving example, not how we can show how much we hate hatred. It's the difference between fighting *for* what we love and fighting *against* what we hate. (And yes, I wrote this long before *The Last Jedi* hit theaters.) I suspect we need a balance of both, but I feel inclined to strive for the first more than the second. Actually, that's not true. I'm significantly more inclined to fight against what I hate rather than for what I love, but I feel strongly that I should try to do the opposite.

As such, I want to promote peaceful and respectful dialogue though I find myself sucked into the mire of political arguments frequently. I know as well as anyone how difficult it can be to keep a civil tone, for there are important issues and serious consequences at stake. But when I stoop to personal attacks, stating my own views as facts or stating facts haughtily as if knowing them makes me a better human somehow, Jesus is not proud of me for being right. When I seek to show that I am right and others are wrong—rather than gain a better understanding of other views, challenge them with honest questions, and respectfully share my own beliefs and the path that led me to hold them—I do not show the rest of the world what it means to follow Christ's teaching and example. When I and so many Christians spew hatred at one another over politics, it makes us a vale of shadows to be avoided, not a light on a hill to be sought.

It all starts with forgiveness. I need to forgive anyone I disagree with if I am to interact with them properly. That sounds sanctimonious, as if by default those I don't agree with are committing some wrong against me, but in a lot of ways that is my default assumption. When someone says something I find hateful, offensive, or personally attacking, I need to first forgive them so my heart doesn't burn against them, destroying any chance of a constructive interaction. When I disagree with someone about my right to healthcare, I need to forgive them, even as I believe firmly that those who don't recognize my right to healthcare don't care about lives like mine and need to be held accountable for the damage they might do to the most vulnerable citizens and to our healthcare system. It's hard to know what that kind of forgiveness looks like, though.

In the context of the church, forgiveness means I need to extend God's grace to my siblings in Christ more. It means no matter how deep my ideological differences with another Christian may go, no matter how profoundly we may disagree about what it means to be part of society and work for good in this world, I don't need to count that against them as a person. When I feel personally attacked by those in the church who would hold me morally accountable for my cancer, or tell me if I had more faith I wouldn't be dealing with it, or support legislation that would erode the patient protection laws that have saved my life during the past few years of expensive medical treatment, I need to forgive them. I need to forgive them for the ways they hurt me as I continue to work against such harmful and toxic views. I don't know exactly what this should look like in my life. But I have some ideas of where to start.

Forgiveness is a conscious choice not to hold a person's actions against them, whether they apologize or even recognize a need to offer an apology. It is essentially waiving our right to use another's actions as leverage against them or as an excuse to retaliate. It doesn't mean everything will go back to the way it was. It doesn't mean we have to forget what the other person did. But it does mean we cannot hate them for their actions, no matter how much we might hate their actions. Forgiveness means, in short, that I must treat all people with equal dignity as image-bearers of God, whether or not I agree with their theology or politics—or whether or not they agree with mine.

Toward the Christians who vocally support repeals of the healthcare laws that have prevented my treatment from being cut off for being too expensive, I must also choose to act this way. Be they voters who supported candidates calling for patient protection law repeals or the legislators themselves who champion this "cause," they are still people made in the image of God. They might be the closest thing I have to enemies, but even (and especially) so, I must love them and pray for them. I have not and am not, so I must start there.

The church is doing wonderful things. I've seen the church at its absolute worst and very best during my cancer treatments, and it's past time now to talk about the best. It's time to explore the greatest parts of what the church is and can be. A critique is only useful if, after you point out areas for improvement, you explore and praise the strengths as well, giving guidance on what to do better and encouragement for what to keep doing well. So I'll do that here, starting with what I hope the church can become.

The church first and foremost should be a family. It doesn't have to get along, and frankly it shouldn't always. My immediate family is reasonably abnormal in that we rarely hide our feelings for the sake of family peace. We all have opinions and we make them known. We call each other out and we voice disagreements whenever they arise. We aren't the most peaceful family, but we aren't artificial either. I wouldn't have it any other way. My hope for the Church is that we can someday grow to become more like that—able to argue amongst ourselves while never doubting the ties of love binding us together as one.

I think sometimes we forget this as a church family. Sometimes we feel that our disagreements are unbridgeable divides. Sure, once in a while they might be, but far more often we simply haven't tried to make a bridge or even find suitable sites for foundations on both sides of the gap. The more we look around at the church in America today, the more it seems that divisions loom everywhere, dividing us into ever-smaller factions. What most of us seem to forget is that disagreement is not always the real issue. It is a profound failure to disagree respectfully and a lack of willingness to learn from disagreement that create a far more severe problem.

When we respectfully and humbly acknowledge whatever truth others may impart while stating that we disagree with the rest of their statements, everyone benefits.

When I've seen this at work in the church, it has been beautiful. I've had my own opinions and the rationale behind my beliefs challenged more constructively by honest, respectful questions than by anything else, and when I can remember to ask respectfully why someone holds to a viewpoint I don't agree with, I feel like I actually get to explain in return where I'm coming from, even as I consider the wisdom the other person has to offer.

None of the ways I've been blessed by the church during my sickness are particularly newsworthy, at least not in our culture where sensationalism and controversy fuel national interest. The small, personal good the

church does every day, like giving extra to those who fall ill or serving meals
to those without adequate food, will never make national headlines. And in
a lot of ways this is exactly how the church should serve others: personally,
locally, genuinely. These real, noble, and wonderful ways that the church is
working for good in this country and the world too often go overlooked.
Sometimes we lose sight of all the good the church is accomplishing.

I owe a lot to the churches that I've been a part of. I know I wouldn't
be who I am without their influences in my life. I grew up in a rather
academic church, attended by professors and (predominately graduate)
students from the University of Notre Dame and Bethel and Saint Mary's
colleges. This church wasn't academic in the sense that it was impersonal
or that the Christian faith was portrayed as some theoretical or speculative
consideration, but it was an intellectually vibrant community that I grew
up thinking was normal. People like Alvin Plantinga went to my church,
and it wasn't until I was ten or twelve that I realized he was perhaps the
preeminent living Christian philosopher. As a kid, I knew him simply as
"Al," a nice guy at church who talked to my Sunday school once about rock
climbing and grace.

Looking back, I see now how my church environment fostered in me a
desire for a greater intellectual understanding of God, as well as an appreciation for robust sermons. In many ways, it is because of my church in
South Bend, Indiana, that I learned to grow from my doubts, ask the kinds
of questions I find fascinating and faith-deepening, and to enjoy enter-
taining the possible answers I find helpful. As far as I'm concerned, you
can't grow up going to church with philosophers and not become keenly
interested in the deeper questions of Christianity. This has held true for me,
and I remain deeply grateful for ways this church fostered in me an abiding
love for the intellectual side of Christianity that has saved me from a crisis
of faith more than once.

The churches I went to while in college and attend now have formed
me in important ways too. Both in the Anabaptist tradition, these Brethren
in Christ and Mennonite churches have helped me grow in my understanding of what it means to live simply and to live differently because of
my faith without becoming irrelevant or absurd to the rest of the world. At
these churches, I've found that it's not about visibly denying yourself the
luxuries, comforts, and ways of the world in an effort to be set apart from
it, as some insist. But neither is it about dismissing that idea and living no
differently—except perhaps on Sunday morning—than anyone else lives.

What I've found in these churches is a way of thinking that captures what I believe a Christ-like life should look like. Following Christ means trying to live a life that runs counter to our materialistic consumer culture in ways that don't necessarily look different on the outside but feel different on the inside. It might mean making do with less, and it might mean buying ourselves the very best we can afford. It depends on the circumstances and the reasons we hold in our hearts for doing so. It means not judging others for the way we perceive their life choices, and asking others to do the same for us. Only in the last few years have I felt that I truly understand what it means to follow Christ in the way I interact with the broader culture I'm a part of.

These churches in the Anabaptist tradition have also given me a greater understanding of my citizenship in heaven and how to regard that first and foremost. I've never been a part of an overtly nationalistic, patriotic church, so I've never been especially tempted to regard the United States as God's chosen country or equate Christianity with patriotism or membership in any particular political party. But I have on occasion visited churches with American flags up front, and as a child I had plenty of friends who held such views, so I'm not ignorant about Christian nationalism. The emphasis of the Mennonite church I attend now seems especially relevant today as Christian nationalism in this country grows stronger. What it means to regard citizenship in heaven above my citizenships in the US and Canada, and what it means to work for God's realm rather than any one political entity here on earth, has helped me as I deal with the deepening mire of the current political landscape. It is this balance of furthering God's realm—inherently political work—while not being swept up in nationalism, demagoguery, or blind partisan loyalty that I think I most appreciate about the Anabaptist tradition.

One final way I've seen the church function wonderfully is how it stays strong across time and space. I grew up in the same church in South Bend, Indiana, for eighteen years, returning occasionally after that when I was home on breaks from college and once during my cancer treatment. It has always been and in some ways may always be my primary church family. When I went back there in summer 2016, it was as if I had never left. I think in many ways I hadn't. I know I have continually been thought of and prayed for by so many there. I have never left their hearts, nor have they left mine. I cannot help thinking that this provides an excellent example of church at its best. It scarcely matters how far away I live or how long it has been between visits. This group of Christians will always be family.

And that's what church can be and should strive to be more often: family. Church is, if nothing else, a big, loud, sometimes obnoxious, sometimes inexpressibly loving family. I'm glad I'm a part of it, even if sometimes it drives me up the wall.

Chapter 8

(Dis)Abilities

After my second round of radiation therapy, I had a couple weeks off for recovery, though I didn't really need them. I was scheduled to start maintenance chemotherapy, a combination of three drugs that should help keep my cancer in check without having so many difficult side effects. I got an extra week off when one of my new drugs didn't get approved by our insurance company right away. So, with Christina's sister visiting us again, now on summer break from teaching, we went to Six Flags Great Adventure in New Jersey, a park I've wanted to visit since 2005 when they built what was at the time the tallest and fastest roller coaster in the world. It's still the tallest though it's been surpassed in speed by a ride in Dubai. More impressive and fun in my opinion is the world's tallest drop ride, a 415-foot free fall that provides a single jolt of adrenaline during its three-second plummet that is unlike anything else I've ever experienced. Sometimes people say cancer treatment is like a roller coaster, but I don't identify with that analogy at all. I love roller coasters. And they follow a set layout.

Once the insurance approval finally went through, I started my new regimen of chemotherapy. One of the biggest changes was doing this chemo in Corning rather than New York City. It made me nervous at first since Memorial Sloan Kettering is a world-renowned cancer center with an oncologist and surgeons who know DSRCT as well as can be hoped for, given its rareness, and I'd had all my treatment there so far. I wasn't sure how I felt about going anywhere else, about seeing a new oncologist, and especially about being anywhere but Sloan Kettering if complications arose.

My apprehension proved needless. The skill and care of the people in Corning, coupled with their willingness to communicate with and take direction from my doctors in New York City, made treatment at home work well. It didn't make much sense to go to New York City one day a week for chemotherapy infusions when it could be done fifteen minutes from home. After the first day, I forgot my uncertainty, and now, years after I started my maintenance chemo, I remain confident that this was the right choice. One of my favorite nurses works at the hospital in Corning, and Christina and I are both glad for her care and friendship.

Maintenance chemotherapy was the same routine for more than a year. I took a chemo pill every night with a snack before bed, and every Wednesday for three weeks I went to the cancer center in Corning, got my port accessed for a couple of hours, and received my chemo infusions. Then I got de-accessed and headed home. I had one week off from infusions between cycles, but I still took the nightly chemo pill during the off weeks. That made it feel less like true time off from chemo in my mind, but fortunately I never noticed any side effects from these pills alone.

I wasn't sure what to expect when I started maintenance chemo. It was supposed to be easy and tolerable, but as my oncologist regularly reminded me with any type of treatment, "Everyone handles it differently." There's no way to know how you'll feel on a chemotherapy regimen until you're on it. Given how terrible my first chemotherapy was, and how tolerable and easy it was expected to be, I was apprehensive, a bit worried that this too would prove difficult.

Thankfully, maintenance chemotherapy was the most tolerable of all the chemo regimens I've been through thus far. For the first few months I felt totally fine, and the only real sign that I was actually on chemo were mouth sores and mildly thinning hair. I soon figured out that Bioètne mouthwash solved the first problem, and I don't care how my hair looks as long as it feels comfortable, which is evidenced by how silly my hair looks most of the time. It got pretty thin by six months into this chemo regimen, but I prefer looking like I'm in the beginning stages of male-pattern baldness to a sunburned scalp or the chill of the wind on my bald head, so I left it alone. I don't have to look at it, after all. Wearing winter hats in the middle of July because it's breezy out and my bald scalp gets cold is annoying. I did it my first year of treatment, and it's fine in the grand scheme of things, but nonetheless I still prefer a little natural insulation and protection from the sun to always needing a hat.

For the first several cycles of maintenance I didn't feel sick, even on the days when I received chemo infusions. I felt marginally more tired than I would have otherwise, but not significantly enough to interfere with life. During one of the first cycles, I was still feeling so well that I even had chemo on the day I left with my dad and sisters on a three-night camping and Six Flags trip in New Jersey and Massachusetts. That first summer of maintenance chemo, when it had not yet started to make me feel chemo-y, I went to a few more theme parks a few more times. I was able to spend a weekend camping and enjoying Cedar Point in Ohio with some childhood friends, Six Flags in New Jersey several more times with a few friends from college, and Six Flags in Montreal when my dad, one of my uncles, and I spent a weekend there for the Formula One Grand Prix. I started following F1 the first year of my cancer treatment since I wanted a sport to watch during the summer when I didn't feel well enough to do much else. Baseball, as fun as it is to go to games in person, isn't something I enjoy on TV. Formula One more than covers the offseason for the NHL and the Premiere League, and I've long had an interest in cars, so it fit the bill of what I was looking for. It also made me much more excited to get radiation since the mold I lay in for those treatments used the same technology they employ for seat fitting in F1.

Maintenance chemotherapy gradually turned more difficult as time progressed. I started to feel weird, then gross, then outright sick on the days I got my infusions. Sometimes I could sleep it off with a nap after getting back home from the hospital, and sometimes those feelings lingered throughout the day. Then they started spilling over to the next day and even two days afterward. Sometimes I got headaches too, though they were manageable with Tylenol.

In October 2016, Christina and I were able to travel to Vancouver, British Columbia, during an off week from chemo to see my dad's side of the family. Several of my aunts and uncles, a cousin, and my Oma— my Dutch grandmother—live in the Vancouver area. They have all been supportive and generous to us, and it was great to be able to visit with them. My oldest sister, Elyssa, also flew out there at the same time to run a half-marathon, and we watched the finish in beautiful Stanley Park.

We enjoyed several more of the sights and activities in and around Vancouver, spending a day in Seattle and another in Whistler where we were able to watch the Canadian luge and bobsled teams practicing up close. Our favorite outing was a visit to the George C. Reifel bird sanctuary on Westham Island. Even without the impressive diversity and sheer number of birds, which I personally loved, the views of the entire area were well worth the trip. From the observation tower, we enjoyed everything from the massive and snowy Mount Baker to the ocean to the often-shrouded North Shore Mountains on the edge of the Vancouver metropolitan area.

All told, it was a wonderful trip and a much-needed break from the monotonous slog of chemo. Even with this relatively easy regimen, I felt worse and worse each infusion day as the cycles added up. My blood counts never dropped to dangerously low levels, but they never got especially high either, and most of my numbers like neutrophil, lymphocyte, and hemoglobin counts held steadily in the lower end of what's acceptable for the last six months or so of this chemo. One of the few numbers that hardly ever went low during any of my treatments was my platelet counts, which have continued to be high ever since I had my spleen removed as part of my first major abdominal surgery. One chemo treatment caused my platelets to drop significantly and necessitated transfusions, but mostly my platelets have stayed high. Among other functions, the spleen filters old and wearing-down platelet cells, so it makes sense that the count remained high. For a little while immediately following my splenectomy, my platelet counts were so high that I was in danger of developing blood clots, but the level balanced out in a month or so and hasn't been an issue since.

The worsening side effects of maintenance chemotherapy began to make other areas of my life more difficult. For example, I wrote most of this chapter the day after more infusions of maintenance chemo. That meant typing it in the bathroom as an email to myself on my phone during an intense, four-hour bout of constipated diarrhea, which was the least pleasant side effect of that chemo and one of the more uncomfortable conditions I know of. Imagine the unpleasant cramping, bloating, feverish chills, and urgency of diarrhea combined at times or alternating in waves with the cramping, bloating, and inability to have a BM of constipation, multiply that by three, and you get an idea of what it's like to have constipated diarrhea. At times like those, I wished for my ileoostomy bag back, even as I appreciated not needing it anymore.

I also became increasingly fatigued as I got through more and more rounds of this chemo. I started to need naps more afternoons than not, and I didn't have the same level of energy as before. Even so, I was still doing better than I had through most of my treatment. I was able to go skiing and snowboarding over Christmas, and I could play hockey, albeit for short shifts with a low-key, non-contact pickup group in town. I'd play until my vision started to go spotty, then I'd spend a few minutes on the bench recovering. It was wonderfully exhausting to play hockey again. I was as active as I could be during this period of maintenance chemo, which was far more so than I had been throughout most of my treatment the previous year. However, I wasn't able to be nearly as active as I was BC, *before cancer*.

My fluctuating activity levels got me thinking about *ableism*—a term I encountered only after my diagnosis and which means discrimination or prejudice against people with disabilities.

I don't know what to think about my physical shape. I'm worn down from more than four years of cancer treatment—there's no doubt about that. What isn't so clear to me is how I should view this fact. How much grace do I need to give myself, how much do I need to simply accept my new and increasing physical limitations? How much do I need to fight them and work to get back in shape as my body will allow? I don't know if there are easy answers to these questions, but in considering them I've discovered a shocking amount of ableism in my own thoughts, even though the last couple of years have revealed to me a horrifying prevalence of ableism in the world around me.

My experiences with cancer quickly revealed my own ableist ideas. Becoming "disabled" as far as the Social Security Administration is concerned started me on this path of discovery. At the start of my treatment, when my oncologist signed the paperwork saying that my health and treatment needs would preclude me from working for at least a year and I became officially "disabled," I wondered about what it really means to be disabled and what our society considers disabled. Apparently, one definition of being able-bodied is the ability to secure a paying job. By such a standard, I was suddenly disabled, thanks to all the chemotherapy, radiation, and surgeries I would need. Yet physically I was unchanged. I didn't feel disabled then, and it took a long time before I considered myself disabled. I thought of myself as less-abled, perhaps. But to claim more than that felt disrespectful to people who have experienced much more significant physical and mental challenges than I have for far longer than a couple of years.

Before I had cancer I thought disabilities were static, permanent conditions. I thought disabilities required the constant use of assistive technologies and aids like wheelchairs or seeing-eye dogs. I thought you had to be "really" disabled for it to count, and I wouldn't have been especially charitable to people in my situation who were classified as disabled. I even considered eyeglasses more as a fashion statement than a piece of assistive technology. I didn't understand the complexity and degrees of disability, and I'd never considered the idea that it could cover a spectrum or range, or that disabilities could fluctuate day by day or month to month.

Until I started hospice (rather than potentially curative treatments), I also did not want to accept myself being disabled. Not forever. Throughout my cancer treatments I always hoped to not have cancer someday, to not have the disabilities that come with my cancer and its treatments; however, tempered with that hope have been the realities of this disease and the knowledge that I simply would not become cancer-free with today's medicine. I also didn't want to accept unnecessary limits. I wanted to give myself the grace not to do what I couldn't do, but I also wanted to push myself to walk more and be active and keep from growing weaker than I need to, even if there were days when I cannot do more than rest.

On the one hand, I needed to remember that I'd been through four years of hellish cancer treatment and give myself some grace about my physical condition. On the other hand, though, if I never pushed myself to recover from surgery, if I didn't try to walk and be active as much as I could every day, I would be letting myself linger in a weaker state of health than necessary. I don't know what the ideal balance might have been, if there even was one. Now, on hospice, it's become a virtual non-issue and I think I can accept any new physical limits that I must, but it's still a difficult balance to know how active to force myself to be each day.

When there was a chance that I might someday become free of cancer, I had harder questions to figure out. I never quite knew how to accept that I would always need a bathroom far more frequently than before, or that due to one of the chemotherapy drug's effects on my heart, I would never be able to lift more than forty pounds safely. I also didn't want to accept my lung capacity decreasing by half or my legs growing weaker—or anything but trying to be in good shape to the best of my abilities.

Most of us use the ableist phrase "good shape." It implies that a higher level of physical fitness is good and a low one is bad. Again, I don't quite know what to think about this dichotomy. It is good to take care of ourselves and strive to be as fit and healthy as our bodies will allow. But it is also ableist to declare that someone who can run a marathon is in "good" shape while someone who can't is in "bad" shape. Surely there's a better term. Regardless of the language we use concerning physical abilities, my experiences with cancer have definitely opened my eyes to ableism.

During my cancer treatment, I've had days when I wished for a wheelchair to use and then immediately chided myself for not being grateful that I *didn't* need one. Then I wondered why I felt that reflexive, self-corrective urge. What is wrong with using a wheelchair when I need one or can benefit from one? Am I too proud? Or am I simply trying to push myself physically so I can recover more quickly from my latest surgery? Is there a part of me that has viewed people who use wheelchairs as somehow lesser, something I don't want to be? Or have I worried too much about what people will think when they see a reasonably healthy-looking young man who is fully capable of walking—albeit not for long—using a wheelchair?

I can't answer questions like these. I've heard that we as a society need to regard equipment like wheelchairs or canes the way we do reading glasses— use them when you need them, and don't use them when you don't. I like that idea, though I know we're far from adopting it.

Beyond the murkiness in my mind, I've discovered a world of ableism, thanks largely to my new and increasing physical limits. Idioms like "stand up for what's right" gained new meaning for me on days when I could barely rise out of bed after a surgery. So too did our tradition of standing to sing at least some of the songs during a church service; I knew I would be far too light headed if I stood up suddenly, especially if I tried to sing rather than merely breathe deliberately and deeply. I've always known that it was kind to say, "All who are able, please stand," but I never realized how important it is until I got cancer. As my physical limitations have increased the longer I've been on cancer treatment, I've become more aware of a range of manifestations of ableism, from our language to our thoughts to our built environment, which doesn't feature nearly enough easy access to bathrooms, ramps, and benches.

If you go through life without having to consider your health or physical abilities, it's easy to take them for granted. And in some ways, I'm inclined to think people should. No one should live in constant fear that their health will change and their physical abilities will become limited. We ought to appreciate our good health and physical abilities, but at the same time, doing this too much can lead to the idea that life without robust health and physical ability is inherently worse in value or quality. Also, when we never consider our health and physical abilities, we ignore the realities of life for those who might not share our way of experiencing the world. We risk being inconsiderate of those whose abilities differ from ours, and we further marginalize those who are already pushed to the periphery by society.

There's a healthy way to balance these ideas and to appreciate health without stigmatizing illness and disability, but I think we rarely see it done well. Instead, ableism commonly takes two forms in our society, often at the same time. First, there is the notion that people with disabilities are somehow lesser people than those without. This form of ableism attaches value to the perceived utility of other people, that is, whether we think they can serve a function we find useful. It's an idea that I reject utterly. Human value comes not from people's abilities or perceived usefulness. Our value is inherent as beings fashioned in the image of God, whatever our particular gifts, talents, and abilities may be. Fortunately, this kind of ableism is condemned whenever people are aware of it, even if it isn't especially well recognized.

In a second, less recognizable and more insidious form of ableism, people take too much pride in their abilities. This second form often goes hand in hand with the most common manifestation of the first, which is attaching too much fear or perceived difficulty to the prospect of becoming disabled.

The first kind of ableism might be easier to recognize in its most egregious form, but it's still pervasive. It's the kind of ableism that asks questions like "Would you rather be blind or deaf?" and debates which would be worse, which would ruin one's life more. Such questions are an insult to those with deafness, blindness, or both, but they also feed the stigma that having such a disability would end life as we know it.

I don't propose taking this idea to the other extreme and ignoring the way disabilities make life more difficult for people, especially those for whom our built environment is not designed. But I don't think we're in any danger of that today. Instead, I think many of us think it's impossible for a person with a disability to live a fulfilling, productive life—and if they do, that life is somehow inspirational.

Indeed, many people living with disabilities are seen not as people but as "inspirations," coping so well with what must be terribly difficult, doing much better than we would if we, God forbid, ever found ourselves knocked down to their lowly position. I've experienced this at times, and while I know the people who say such things mean well and seek to be encouraging, I cannot help feeling patronized when people tell me I'm dealing well with my cancer—*so much better than they would in my shoes*—and how I'm inspiring and my terrible situation makes their difficulties seem trivial by comparison. If I can help bring perspective to someone's life and inspire them, that's great, but I wish I could to this without being made to feel like little more than inspiration porn, a story to be consumed and an interesting side show, not a person with whom to interact.

I don't have a perfect solution to this problem, and I'm sure a part of how I feel about it depends on my mood. Hearing how inspiring I am as I deal with cancer might be exactly what I need to hear sometimes, and it might annoy me at other times depending on what I've been going through and how well I believe I'm handling it. My advice would be for people not to worry to the point that they don't say anything or avoid people with disabilities because they're afraid of saying the wrong thing. Instead, I encourage people to acknowledge that serious illness is a tricky situation, to be willing to apologize if they unintentionally cross lines, and to try to be present and meet the person where they are. I wish I had a better answer or more specific advice, but I don't think there's a formula for treating people with dignity. See and respond to the person instead of to the illness or disability. Just be kind.

It's easy to credit ourselves too much for our abilities and good health. I know that's true for me. This kind of ableism ties in closely with more standard ableism, since crediting ourselves for our health and abilities pairs easily with blaming others for their illnesses or disabilities. But it also stands alone sometimes, and we see it when people give too much credit to their diet or workout routine for their health and wellness.

I've encountered one other unhealthy view of human ability while going through cancer treatment: I think sometimes we Christians are too quick to discount our own abilities. Sometimes we declare things that are difficult to be beyond our ability to influence, so we turn them over to God. It's important to recognize our limits and our dependence on God, but too often I see this used as an excuse for inaction. Sometimes, this is a way to shirk responsibility under the guise of reliance on God. God gives us abilities and talents and expects us to use them. When we don't, we dishonor God and achieve less than God wants of us.

In extreme cases, this can look like forgoing medical treatment in favor of God's healing. I alluded to this idea in chapter 4 when I covered the subject of prayer, and now I'd like to expand on it. As I said earlier, it's okay to believe in a God of healing and to ask God to heal us, but if that's all we do, if we do not also use our intellect and knowledge, we miss out on many of the channels God has provided for us to find healing.

If we spurn the knowledge and care of modern medicine, choosing instead to rely on God alone, we, in fact, rely less on God. If knowledge comes from God, that includes knowledge of the human body and the vastly complicated ways in which it works and can be healed. To trust fully in God is to trust also in our own abilities, in the talents, knowledge, and skills that God has bestowed upon us. Modern medicine and prayers for healing can work together, and successful medical treatment can be an answer to prayer just as much as a healing miracle. There aren't many people today who claim we should forgo modern medicine in favor of prayer alone when it comes to physical health, but this strain of theological malpractice is common in discussions about mental health, especially with depression and anxiety. I've not had mental illness, so I haven't experienced this idea directed at me, but I've seen it enough to know that it bears mentioning here. Physical health and mental health both require care beyond faith and prayers. They both require trained professionals, specialists who know how to help, medicine, therapists of all kinds, and more.

Prayer can and should work in tandem with modern medicine, and we can never go wrong praying that the medical professionals treating us have the wisdom and presence of mind needed to treat us as best they can. As with the subject of "thoughts and prayers" I discussed earlier, it's a balance. We should be wary of relying too much on our own abilities—leading to unhealthy views of our worth or accomplishments—while striving to use our abilities as best we can.

Chapter 9

Advent

Every six to eight weeks during my maintenance chemotherapy, I had another set of scans. Every couple months or so, we'd take a Corporate Angel flight into New York City and I'd head to the pediatric floor to get my port accessed and have blood work done. Then I'd go down to the imaging department and spend an hour reading, tweeting, and drinking more contrast. I've gotten good at drinking the stuff, though I stand by my assessment in chapter 1 that it tastes worse the more you drink. The hardest part of scans, though, is usually lying still for up to an hour. Sometimes it's easy. Sometimes I fall asleep and it's over before I know it. Other times I need to go to the bathroom about three minutes in. I probably wouldn't have to go if I were to spend that same forty-five minutes to an hour at home with a bathroom just a few steps away. But the knowledge that I have to hold it and lie still makes doing those things all but impossible.

My scans during this time continued showing spots of suspicion and interest. Some of them came and went, and some of them stayed steady or grew slowly worse. By early 2017, I was growing frustrated and ready to try something else if my next scan results showed any growth at all. In February, they did, and before I even voiced my opinion and desire to try a more aggressive approach, my incredible surgeon proposed a couple of surgeries to go in and remove everything that was lighting up suspiciously. At this point, I had four spots of interest in my chest and three in my abdomen.

First, I had another laparoscopic chest surgery to remove the suspicious areas in my chest. It went fine, and about half of the spots tested positive for DSRCT, the rest being nothing more than normal lymph nodes. Recovery did not go so easily, though. For the first time in my cancer treatment, I experienced complications from a surgery.

The chest tube they had to leave in after this surgery continued to drain for several days until suddenly it stopped because the drain clogged somewhere inside me, leaving the fluid to build up in my chest. In the course of an evening, breathing grew increasingly difficult and my oxygen saturation began to fluctuate. I went back onto supplemental oxygen and forced myself to draw slow, steady breaths, breaths that were much too shallow. It felt like breathing against a brick wall. My lungs fought for every bit of space to expand, but it wasn't nearly enough. They tried injecting a solution into the drain tube to clear it out, but it didn't work. So I had another drain put in with local anesthetic.

More than two liters flowed out of my chest in about fifteen minutes. Suddenly, I had space in my chest again for my lungs to expand, and that hurt more than the fluid had. My lungs felt like rubber bands stretched to their limits, like balloons being inflated to the point of bursting, like a charley horse and a pulled muscle at the same time. The sudden extra space to breathe felt like too much for my lungs, which seemed to have gotten used to working in limited, fluid-filled space overnight. But that pain passed quickly, and soon I was breathing easier again. The problem was that I still had to deal with the fluid.

We tried an interventional radiology procedure to inject dye into my lymphatic system, map out where the leak might be in my chest, and hopefully seal it up, but it didn't work. The sedatives I was on for this procedure made me combative and angry, and apparently I swore fluently at everyone and demanded to go back to my hospital room and a more comfortable bed. If I could apologize to the people from that IR team, I would.

Since this procedure wasn't able to find and stop the leak of lymphatic fluid into my chest, I needed yet another surgery. The hope was to do it laparoscopically, using the same four small spots to enter my thoracic cavity, but there was also a chance that they would need to perform a thoracotomy to find and stop the leak. That is what happened, so I woke up with a long incision following the curve of my right shoulder blade. My back, shoulder, and upper arm were profoundly sore for quite a while. It took probably six months to get to where I had no soreness or pain in my shoulder, but the scar tissue means I have a slightly reduced range of motion in that shoulder. But my dauntless surgeon was at least able to find and clean up the source of leaking in my chest, so the surgery was a success. With two chest surgeries in such a short time came numbness from damaged nerves. This numbness spread across my rib cage and made deep inhalations difficult. The issue has improved significantly, though it involved a long, slow process of strange sensations like pins, needles, bee stings, tingling, and buzzing as the nerves along my ribcage come back to life and regrew.

A couple weeks after that chest surgery, I had another abdominal surgery, the fourth time my largest incision scar has been opened. Three spots were removed, two of which were cancerous. They tried a new radiation technique in which a radioactive fluid dripped over the course of half an hour onto the spots where the cancerous nodes were removed. I'm not a big fan of radiation to my belly, but this method sent targeted radiation to a potential problem area. While the goal of surgery is to get every bit of cancer out, there's always a chance that even one cell might get left behind, and one cell is all it takes.

I had lingering complications from this abdominal surgery as well. It took me more than a week to get out of the hospital, which was made better by watching the entire *Fast and Furious* franchise for the first time, but it was still a difficult wait. I had to work on walking again, first just a few steps, then a full lap of the inpatient floor, then five, then ten laps. I had to work on breathing, trying to inhale more than two liters and failing miserably, though my baseline lung capacity during cancer treatment was more than twice that.

I was out of the hospital for one night before I went right back in, my abdomen painfully full of fluid. I had the fluid drained under local anesthetic, though they didn't leave a drain in since there seemed to be a decent chance that my body would reabsorb whatever fluid might be left. Having a hole punched into my side to drain abdominal fluid while I'm wide awake isn't a procedure I'd care to do again. We waited around a few more days to see if the fluid came back.

It did.

My surgeon came in at 6 a.m. on Easter Sunday to place another drain under local anesthetic, this one draining two liters, much as my chest drain had a couple weeks previously.

This drain stayed in for about a week, after which the draining seemed to have slowed enough that I would be able to reabsorb whatever fluid remained. It became apparent after a couple of days, though, that the drain had clogged, and I soon found my belly full of another two liters. I was back home in Corning by the time this became clear, so I had the fluid drained at the local hospital, which meant removing more than two liters but not leaving a drain in and instead being referred back to New York City for follow up. The fluid built up again, and another two liters or so were drained, this time with heavier sedation, which meant I wasn't nearly as aware of the procedure as it happened and didn't remember it at all within an hour.

To test a new theory, I didn't have the drain left in and I tried drinking extra fluids so I wouldn't need IV hydration. Given my previous bad experience with an interventional radiology treatment—the other course of action my surgeon suggested I try—I wanted to rule out everything else before I did that. So I drank four liters a day and didn't get extra IV fluids with chemo. For a week or so, it seemed that this might be working, that perhaps IV fluid was being absorbed by my body in a weird way and pooling in a spot in my belly that the latest surgery had opened up. But then it became clear that my abdomen was, once again, filling with fluid.

Yet again I went into New York City to get a drain placed. This time, I had it placed under general anesthetic, since I had enough time to plan ahead and not eat beforehand, and I was growing tired of being poked in my stomach so much. I woke up swearing prodigiously after this procedure but in a happy way, which was still a bit odd but much more pleasant than the combative and angry swearing I'd unleashed after the interventional radiology procedure following my chest surgery.

It seemed that interventional radiology was the only course of action left to try, other than opening me up again and trying to find and close the leak by hand, which wasn't an option unless the IR procedure failed, making surgery worth the further toll on my body. So I reluctantly agreed, not having much of a choice at this point and having exhausted every other possible option. I caught a break, though, and the IR procedure worked. They injected the dye into my lymph system and almost immediately found the leak, which they were able to coagulate without a problem. I left my abdominal drain in for another week, wanting to play it safe, but it stopped draining almost instantly.

Thankfully, I haven't had any further complications since I had the drain removed, and the issue of fluid buildup finally seems to be resolved. It took longer to take care of than it should have, in large part due to my unwillingness to try another interventional radiology procedure, but I only say that now in hindsight. At the time, I just didn't want to have to go through another IR procedure like my first one. I chalk it up to burning out a little after more than two years of treatment, or to stubbornness, or to wishful thinking that it would resolve on its own without more poking and prodding. Probably a little of all three.

After these surgeries, I went back into maintenance chemotherapy. In fact, I started it up again well before the abdominal fluid complications were resolved. The cumulative effect of more and more cycles of maintenance chemotherapy combined with ongoing complications and recovery from surgery made this a rough period. By May, a month or so after my last surgery, I was back down to my lowest weight, in the low 150s. I've gained perhaps 15 pounds since then through hard work, dedication, my wife's continuing, loving reminders to EAT EAT EAT, and as much protein-rich food and ice cream as I can manage, but it's still a constant struggle just to maintain weight, much less gain a little.

In fall 2017, I tried a second clinical trial, testing a new drug designed to attack DSRCT through a different pathway than anything I've had previously. This trial was only available in Cleveland, so my wife and I drove five hours and stayed at our first Hope Lodge, which is basically a more cancer-specific Ronald McDonald house for older people. It was a strange change of pace being the youngest person there, but it was a lovely place to stay, within walking distance of the Cleveland Clinic, a gentrified part of town with a bunch of restaurants we love like Qdoba, and multiple museums, though we didn't spend more than a few nights in the city and didn't have time to explore the museums when they were open.

This clinical trial was an easy treatment regimen, just five pills once a week with no side effects. We used the time as a break to go on another road trip, made possible by financial gifts from generous people. As it was the start of October, we decided to skip Glacier National Park since it was too cold. Instead, we headed across South Dakota, stopping at Badlands National Park, Wall Drug—because you kind of have to—and the Black Hills. We made a quick detour to Devil's Tower National Monument before spending a few wonderful, freezing days in Yellowstone, where the elk were bugling and the specks on the edge of a snow bank a mile away were wolves, or so said the people who had been watching them all day. The highlight for me was a pair of bald eagles hunting a duck on the Yellowstone River, working as a team to eventually catch it despite its frequent dives underwater. Nature is cruel, but it is also beautiful and awesome.

After a couple of nights by Jackson Hole, we went to Antelope Island and Salt Lake City in Utah before continuing to Zion National Park. It was so busy that we stayed for free on public lands outside the park, rather than get in line by 5 a.m. for a chance at a campground. We followed that with Bryce Canyon, a nice stop on our way to our next real destination—Grand Staircase Escalante National Monument.

We were alone, it was silent, and it was the most spectacular part of our trip, perhaps in part because I'd never been there before, but mostly because of the lovely time we had there. We searched for (and maybe found?) some dinosaur footprints and spent a while exploring slot canyons, even stumbling across the first tarantula I've ever seen in the wild. (My heart breaks at the recent assault on this monument and neighboring Bears Ears. These are wild, wonderful places that deserve protection even if they weren't sacred land for indigenous people in the area, and even more so *because* of that.)

After our time in Grand Staircase, we detoured to the North Rim of the Grand Canyon on a bit of a whim. That campground was full so we spent another night on public lands just outside the park after watching rangers radio-collar a bison that evening.

We then headed toward Moab and only ended up as far as Page, Arizona. We got a motel since we needed to do laundry and shower after so many days of camping on public lands with only the water we brought with us.

After a look at the dizzying Glen Canyon Dam, we headed onwards through Monument Valley before reaching Moab, Utah, another busy place. All the camping in the region was full, and we had to drive another hour to get lodging. We returned the next day for a quick tour of Arches and Canyonlands National Parks, which were both beautiful but horribly busy, and then we headed out.

A night at the beautiful Colorado National Monument came next, though by this point we'd seen our share of red rocks. We stopped for a short hike in Vail before we made it to the Denver, Colorado, area. We spent a couple of nights there and caught up with one of my childhood friends— the same one I've been to Cedar Point with the last few summers—and my cousin whom I hadn't seen in too many years. We loved Denver and are ready to move there as soon as we're able—like, once my health stops preventing us from doing that sort of thing and we win the lottery.

Next, we stopped in Nebraska to visit my sister Korynne and her then-fiancé/now-husband. We made it from Nebraska back to Waukesha, Wisconsin, in time for my grandmother's surprise birthday party, stopped briefly in Holland, Michigan, to see Christina's grandparents, and then went home to Corning for about two days.

Then Christina was a bridesmaid in her best friend's wedding near Baltimore, Maryland, and we headed from there to Cleveland again for scans and, hopefully, to continue on the clinical trial. It had been a great six weeks, with another once-in-a-lifetime opportunity to travel and see wonderful sights and people. Since my cancer diagnosis, I'd now been lucky enough to have two of these trips.

My next scans showed mixed results, which meant I could stay on the trial, though it wasn't quite what we were hoping for. Six weeks later, I had my next set of scans. I'd been feeling fine, and we started to let ourselves look for places to rent in town, thinking that maybe now we could reasonably expect to live on our own. I even looked for jobs in the area. I had a job at Pizza Hut if I wanted it, and I got all set up to start substitute teaching, since that would allow me to work flexibly.

The clinical trial had been too easy, though. As I said at the time, "It's not having side effects, but that might just mean it isn't having *any* effects," and this ended up being more or less the case. My second scan on this trial showed too much growth of the spots they were tracking, and I couldn't stay on the trial any longer.

I went back to a few more rounds of an intense chemo called doxorubicin that I had taken in 2015, along with a brand-new immunotherapy drug that had just gotten approved. Unfortunately, I'm terribly allergic to it. I actually triggered a code blue during the first infusion, not because I actually stopped breathing but because they needed to get doctors to me ASAP. I sat up thinking I was going to throw up, and then I tried to dive onto the floor since I was light headed, and I barely remember any of it because I was flitting in and out of consciousness the whole time. I also had swelling and hives everywhere. We eventually figured out a regimen of Benadryl, hydroxyzine, Claritin, and something else that allowed me to get the immunotherapy infusions without a hassle. And I kept an EpiPen on standby, just in case.

I hit my lifetime limit for doxorubicin, which is a shame because it held my disease fairly steady for a few months, but at a certain point I'd be risking cardiac damage if I took any more. It's still an option to help me buy a couple more months sometime down the road, but it's more of a last resort. I took some time off to be a "bridesman" in my sister's wedding in April 2018. In May I started Votrient, an oral chemo that I simply took at home and that didn't having many side effects at all, other than sending me to the bathroom a little more often and a lot more urgently. It also turned my hair white, lending my beard a more distinguished, wiser look. In July and August 2018, I tried yet another immunotherapy clinical trial. It carried a lot of side-effects like fevers, headaches, congestion, and more. Through this point, my cancer treatment has involved a lot of waiting for good results that realistically are not likely.

The best-case scenario that I ever really hoped for and worked toward is a prognosis of "no evidence of disease," or NED. NED is the closest I could have ever hoped to come to "cured" or "in remission." They don't use that kind of terminology with cancers like DSRCT. The best we could have hoped for is that, as far as we can tell, there is no evidence to suggest that I have cancer actively growing in me. It's kind of like aliens. Seeing them will prove they exist, but not seeing them will never disprove their existence. NED means that we don't see any cancer, but it isn't definitive proof that we aren't overlooking it and it's hiding somewhere. I never achieved NED, and I now will never get there, but that was the goal for the better part of four years of treatment. NED is the best I could ever (un?)realistically hope for. Not a cure, not a certain guarantee of health, just a lack of evidence that I have any cancer left. For a long time, my cancer was a chronic condition, managed and kept in check but still very much there. That runs counter to how most of us usually think about cancer, myself included.

In American culture we like to have two simple options. Things are either true or false, good or bad, or some other simple dichotomy. We often see black and white when a full spectrum of colors lies in between, and we fail to appreciate ranges of possibilities. I realized this on a deeper level when I experienced how often people thought of cancer as something that either is being treated or has been cured, as if those were the only two options for a person still living after a cancer diagnosis.

After I finished radiation, the last of my planned courses of treatment, it was difficult to explain that I didn't know whether or not I was done with treatment. I had finished everything planned, but my scans weren't definitively clear and I ultimately ended up doing another three years of treatment, and counting. Throughout my treatment, I didn't have any idea what an end to my treatment would look like. Even if I did get a scan result showing no evidence of disease, I would still likely do more treatment of some sort. I'd stay on whatever has the best chance of keeping me NED as long as I could. If I'd ever gotten to no evidence of disease, I'd likely have done more maintenance chemotherapy just to be safe, potentially for years. I don't know how I'd convince myself to keep going through more of this after getting a clear scan, but I also know it would be foolish to stop everything at the first NED result only to have a relapse because I didn't feel like sticking it out another month or two.

And even if I did decide to stop everything with the first NED scan result, I would still need more follow-up scans, probably every three months at first, then every six, then annually. Beyond that, there's no protocol, since hardly anyone gets that far with DSRCT, but I'd still be years away from being totally free from cancer and the medical procedures it necessitates. I would also still need to take a handful of pills daily to combat the toll my treatment has taken on my immune system. I might not need all of my antibiotics and antivirals if I stop treatment completely, but that could take a while and I really don't know. Realistically, I'll be on at least penicillin for the rest of my life. Even under the best possible circumstances, I wouldn't be clearly done with cancer-related medical procedures and prescriptions for a long time.

Rare as my cancer might be, I'm hardly the only one with this kind of experience regarding the end of treatment. My friend who, as I mentioned earlier, went to basketball games at Madison Square Garden during his chemotherapy, didn't enjoy an especially clear divide between being in treatment and being done with it. Six months after he finished his planned treatment, he had surgery to replace the titanium femur he had received the previous year but now had worked itself loose somehow. Recently, he underwent yet another surgery to shore up the prosthetic femur and tighten some screws. While most people wouldn't consider either surgery a part of "cancer treatment" itself, it is only because he had osteosarcoma in his leg that most of his femur had to be replaced with titanium. These surgeries were in many ways a part of his cancer treatment even though he had been declared NED half a year before and remains, thankfully, clear of his cancer today.

For many of us, cancer treatment becomes uncertain once the planned course of treatment ends. Achieving NED can happen multiple times, with recurrences interrupting everything and wreaking havoc on the lines between "cancer patient" and "cancer survivor." When dealing with aggressive cancers, it is nearly impossible to find an exact end point to treatment. Treatment sort of slowly ends without any fanfare.

Given what I had seen of cancer prior to 2015, I would never have dreamed that the waters would be so murky at the end of planned treatment. That's not what you see on TV or online. Videos of patients dancing on their last day of chemo or ringing a bell to declare themselves cured are far more palatable and therefore popular than the unsatisfying end to treatment that people like me often have. Also, the weeks immediately following my last day of originally planned treatment—radiation—were far worse than the weeks leading up to them, and I wouldn't have felt like celebrating even if I had thought I was done forever with cancer treatment. It's little wonder then why people don't hear much about this kind of experience with finishing cancer treatment. We like closure. We like to mark the moment when one has moved from being in treatment to being cured. We like simple options, not the complex decisions and uncertainties that many of us with difficult cancers face.

Living the realities of an uncertain cancer with no clear end in sight seems worse than it actually is, though. I'm not saying it's fun or easy, but it's not so different from anything else in life that's beyond our control. When I have a scan, my wife and I hope for the best, remember the possibility of the worst, and honestly don't think about it much at all, choosing instead to enjoy the time we have rather than agonize over upcoming results. There is always time to deal with the results, whatever they might be, once they come in. Worrying about them won't influence them. Sometimes putting aside all thoughts of the impending scan results is nearly impossible, but that's where distractions like video games like come in. My heart still skips a beat when the phone rings while we're expecting scan results, but at least it isn't racing all day—only when a creeper blows up something I spent an hour building in Minecraft. Having a small thing like the hostile mobs of Minecraft to worry about and distract me from the disquietude of looming, potentially life-changing scan results helps me. As I've said, I like to sweat the small stuff.

During my cancer treatment, my future has been determined scan-by-scan. Christina and I waited for conclusively cancer-free results for years though we knew we most likely wouldn't ever see them. We awaited scan results we didn't expect to get, scarcely daring to hope for the good news we desperately desired. In a lot of ways, all this waiting felt like a morbid version of Advent.

Advent—those weeks leading up to Christmas—is a season of waiting. And a lot of times it feels like I've done more waiting than anything else the past few years. I've waited for my initial biopsy results, waited for blood work results, waited for my urine to get to the right specific gravity to start chemo, waited for chemo to end, waited for radiation, waited for a clinical trial, waited for surgery again and again and again, waited for relief from shingles, waited for painkillers to kick in, waited for constipation and diarrhea to end, waited for hemorrhoids to heal, waited in waiting rooms for pretty much all of the above, waited for scans to start, waited for scan results. I'm always waiting for my next scans so that I can start waiting for those results. Really, I've been waiting for years for the results we want, for the seemingly unachievable *no evidence of disease* pronouncement.

All that waiting has made me think about the waiting we do during the Advent season. Advent is, after all, about waiting for the arrival of the Messiah, the deliverer who will establish God's kingdom here on earth.

Advent might mean "coming," but for me it has always felt more like "waiting." For me, the best part of the Advent season is the knowledge that, though we wait for Christmas Day to celebrate the birth of Jesus, Christ has already come. God is already here with us. God's kingdom is already among us, existing everywhere we work to spread God's love.

That stands in stark, comforting contrast to the waiting I do for scan results that I don't really expect. I may never get the good news of *no evidence of disease*, but I've already received far better news that makes that okay. During Advent, we wait for a God who enters into the messiness and uncertainty of this world, looking for a tomorrow made better by God's presence in it. In many ways, this seems an especially fitting activity as I wait for definitively clear scans, whether or not I ever get them. I might wait the rest of my life for clear scan results that never come, but at least God is with me through it all.

Closely tied to the season of Advent, a time of waiting for God's arrival here on earth as a human, is the idea of the incarnation, that God became human to share in our experience and do for us what we could not do. I've lived this idea to a tiny degree myself during my time in cancer treatment, and it's renewed my appreciation and furthered my understanding of what the incarnation might mean and signify, both about us and about God.

When we got the diagnosis over four years ago now, I took the news much better than a lot of other people. Better than anyone, honestly. Partly because of my generally carefree nature and the way my diagnosis didn't fly in the face of my beliefs, I also attribute a good part of this to knowing that I, not someone I love, had to go through the hellacious process.

It would be far worse to have to watch someone I care about endure round after round of chemo, surgery followed by surgery, followed by still more surgeries and truly debilitating radiation treatment, followed by more of the same for a second year, then a third year, and finally a fourth year. On the other hand, several people have expressed to me that they wish it were them, not me, going through it all. It is, I think, a natural reaction when we see people we care about suffering. We want to take it from them, to carry their burden and give them some respite from their trials. This is why I would never let someone take my cancer from me and bear it themselves, even if that were possible.

In so many ways, I am grateful that it is me, not other people I know and love, going through this. For one, my body seems to handle the craziness reasonably well, and to look at me now you might never guess what I've gone through the past few years, as long as I keep my shirt on, covering my scars. I'm worn down, certainly, but I'm also doing surprisingly well. I could easily be doing a lot worse. I know that not everyone is so robust or able to handle this without it taking a more serious toll on their bodies and their baseline level of health. I may be down about 50 pounds from where I was before my ordeal began, but it makes me look like a distance runner rather than whatever I looked like before. Couch potato, maybe? But I haven't had any truly serious, dangerously life-threatening side effects from my treatment. That isn't true for a lot of people going through this kind of ordeal. I heal quickly and I've been very fortunate. For that, I am immensely grateful.

My gratitude that it is me and not my wife, siblings, or any number of other people going through this in my place extends well beyond the practicality of how my body has handled it. I sincerely doubt that I would have remained half so calm and happy as I've been this past year were it my wife, not me, going through the miserable treatments. I think that's a significant reason some people have expressed to me that they wish they could have cancer instead of me. And when they do, I'm grateful that they love me enough to want to carry this burden in my place. . . but I think, "Well, that's really sweet, but I'd never let you." I would never let someone take this from me and go through it in my stead. It's so much harder to see a loved one endure something difficult than it is to go through it yourself.

I think that's how God feels. Perhaps for God it was so unbearable to see people muddling through their own mistakes that God came down to go through it all for us, providing us with clearer guidance and giving us a way to be free from our wrongdoings and the suffering they can bring. Much like the people who have expressed that they wished they could take my cancer from me and go through the treatments themselves, God looked at humanity and could not help but become incarnate as a person, go through the human experience of life, and endure the consequences of sin on our behalf. While it's impossible, of course, for any of us to actually take someone else's disease and go through their misery for them, it's comforting to have a God who can do much the same thing, and in fact already did.

Epilogue

About three quarters of the way through writing this book, I realized that I glossed over a bunch of the side effects and difficulties I've dealt with during my grueling cancer treatments, so I'll mention some of the more interesting ones here. I worry that in trying to keep this from becoming a morbid account of one struggle after another, I've painted too sunny a picture of what it means to go through rigorous and aggressive cancer treatment. I want this to be a realistic and honest examination of my experience with cancer, and as such I think it's worth sharing a few of the more significant physical challenges I've faced during the last three years.

I've had numbness from knee to mid-thigh in both of my legs, one at a time, after different abdominal surgeries. Both times it took several months for all my feeling to come back, and as I write this my left leg is still mildly numb in a six-inch swath from my knee upwards. It doesn't affect my mobility and I don't notice it much, but sometimes I get a weird tickle there reminding me of this amusing effect from my cancer treatments.

On the subject of nerves, I also finally began to experience some neuropathy after a year or so of maintenance chemotherapy. Neuropathy is a common side effect for nearly every sort of chemotherapy, and it's a minor miracle that I didn't experience it much earlier and far more severely. As it is, I went through a few months with a little numbness and tingling in my hands and feet, and I still feel it in my toes and the balls of my feet sometimes. It feels like the sensation you get when you first begin to regain feeling after you've sat awkwardly on one of your feet and it goes numb. It's not that bad all things considered, though it is annoying at times. There have been a few days when it started to interfere with my ability to type, which was the most frustrating aspect of this side effect. Thankfully, though, my neuropathy remained mild and intermittent, growing worse by the third week of my maintenance chemo cycle and lessening considerably during my off week. These days, it lingers only mildly in my feet, and I don't notice it often, probably because it's mild and steady enough that I've gotten used to it.

One of the most unpleasant side effects of cancer and its treatment was hemorrhoids, which for me was combined with mucositis from chemotherapy. Mucositis is essentially a breakdown of mucus membranes, which can affect everything from the nose and mouth through the entirety of the digestive tract. As I experienced hemorrhoids in concert with mucositis, they made it feel like I was passing razor blades with each bowel movement. With ten to twenty BMs a day like I had during that phase of treatment, the process became unbearable.

I also got shingles a second time following the election of 2016. I have no doubt that this bout of shingles was brought on by the election results, specifically the sudden uncertainty about the future of our healthcare system and the numerous patient protection provisions that had saved my life. Fortunately, I was much more familiar with the early signs of shingles this time, and I recognized their telltale itchy tingliness right away. I was able to get on an antiviral medication against them just a few hours after I first noticed anything amiss, and they cleared up before becoming bad. I still feel the lingering effects from two separate rounds of shingles, both near each other on the left rear of my head. Sometimes the tingling and itching is so intense that I have to check in a mirror to see if there are any fresh, visible spots. But so far it has been a residual effect, not a new flare up, though it's a long-term consequence of shingles that can last months or even years, sometimes never disappearing completely.

My left leg has mild swelling most days. It has ever since they stopped the leak of my lymph system in my abdomen. At its worst, it makes my leg feel a little sore and less mobile than it would be otherwise, so it isn't too bad.

Recently—as of the summer of 2018—I'm having increasing digestive troubles related to a tumor growing near my pancreas. It makes it hard to eat and hard to digest food.

I have thirteen impressive surgical scars and the pictures to prove them.

I experience physical reminders every day, from frequent, urgent trips to the bathroom ever since my ileostomy takedown to shortness of breath, light-headedness, and a significant decrease in my flexibility and range of motion, especially in my abdomen and chest where I've had multiple surgeries. I cannot escape cancer and the dozens of daily reminders it provides me of my own mortality and capacity to experience suffering.

But as I hope I've made clear throughout this book, cancer does not merely bring pain and suffering, heartbreak and stress, and death. Yes, cancer is horrible. Way too many children have very little hope to reach their next birthday thanks to cancer, and I grieve for them and their families. I have plenty of reason to hate cancer, and I certainly do.

But I would be remiss if I didn't appreciate the many ways cancer—or at least my reaction to it—has enriched my life as well.

The last three years have given me time to see interesting things and have fun. I was able to finish writing the young adult fantasy trilogy I first started when I was fourteen, as well as write this book and a few others for which I'm currently seeking publishers—a fantasy series, some sci-fi, and a young adult utopia (or is it a dystopia?). I've been able to enjoy the best that New York City has to offer, from Central Park to an array of restaurants to numerous world-class museums. I've also been able to enjoy the Corning Museum of Glass far more often than I ever would have without cancer. I've been to a variety of sporting events including my first NFL game, one game each for the Mets and Yankees, a Formula One grand prix, and, best of all, numerous NHL games including a playoff, none of which would have happened if cancer had not shown up in my life. I've enjoyed the Bronx Zoo, Broadway plays, and vacations from Quebec to California and plenty in between for good measure. Cancer has given me time to travel and an excuse to do things I would otherwise have put off for some future day that might never arrive.

But cancer has blessed my life in far more profound ways than just fun activities and amusing pastimes. I have grown closer to my wife, whose unfailing support, love, and kindness have made it worthwhile to keep going on the roughest days. Last May, we celebrated our fifth wedding anniversary shortly after passing the three-and-a-half-year mark since my diagnosis. It's weird that I've had cancer for more than half of our marriage. In some ways, it seems like only a day or two ago that we sat eating Domino's pizza in a Super 8 in New Jersey the evening before my first meeting with the team at Sloan Kettering, not the nearly four years ago that it's actually been. In a lot of ways, it does not feel like more than half our marriage has involved hospitals, surgery, chemo, and more. I suppose that's partly because we knew each other for several years before we got married.

When I look back on the last year and a half, the recollections that come most readily to my mind are not the sickness of chemo and radiation, the pain of recovering from surgery, the side effects of treatment, and the side effects of the drugs taken to reduce those side effects. Rather, I primarily remember more the fun we've had, the memories we've made, the time spent together, and the closeness we've created. The fun and excitement of New York City and our two road trips of a lifetime throughout the American West have given us thousands of fantastic memories together, but even more than these I remember the quiet, normal moments, like sitting and reading in our favorite spot in Central Park or listening to an audiobook together, lying in a hammock on pleasant afternoons in Corning, watching *Parks and Recreation* together when I was too tired to do much else, playing video games while listening to podcasts, writing a blog post or chapter in one of my books while Christina wrote in her journal, or roasting marshmallows around a fire. To make a long story short, it doesn't seem like cancer has taken up more than half our marriage because, quite simply, it hasn't. We haven't let it, as much as has been possible.

While it's negatively affected a lot of things for us, it has also given us more time together than we would have had otherwise and led us to a deeper love for and appreciation of each other and what it means to be partners in this crazy life. For that I am immensely grateful.

Cancer has also nudged me closer to friends outside my family, be they people I've known since before I can remember or those I've only met online. Thanks to cancer, I've made new friends and gotten back in touch with some from long ago. These last three years have served as wonderful reminders of what it means to be rich in relationships and blessed in the elements of life that matter most.

To say it has been the best of times and the worst of times might be a cliché, but it is true. There have been times, however brief, when I was ready to quit. There have been times, far more often than not, when I'd do anything to keep going. Sometimes I absolutely hate cancer, and sometimes I truly love some of what it has done for me. Often both at once. It reminds me of Romans 8:28 and the idea that God works in all things—even and especially the worst things—to bring about good. I certainly owe cancer for my deeper appreciation of life and time spent with loved ones. Cancer has opened my eyes to the depths and heights of human experience and shown me new and more intimate ways of relating to God and understanding God's world. It's not that I needed cancer to learn these lessons, and it's not that I got cancer so that my life could benefit from it in these ways. But cancer has forced me to grow and gain a clearer perspective on life, a deeper relationship with and understanding of God, and better relationships with the people I care about the most. Cancer has given me peace about living and dying. And for those reasons, I am thankful I got cancer . . . even though I wish desperately that I never had.